**HEALTH CARE ISSUES, COSTS AND ACCESS**

# A SYSTEMS ENGINEERING APPROACH TO BETTER, LESS EXPENSIVE HEALTH CARE

# HEALTH CARE ISSUES, COSTS AND ACCESS

Additional books in this series can be found on Nova's website under the Series tab.

Additional e-books in this series can be found on Nova's website under the e-book tab.

HEALTH CARE ISSUES, COSTS AND ACCESS

# A SYSTEMS ENGINEERING APPROACH TO BETTER, LESS EXPENSIVE HEALTH CARE

ADELINE PEATERSON
EDITOR

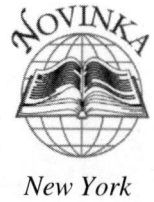

New York

Copyright © 2014 by Nova Science Publishers, Inc.

**All rights reserved.** No part of this book may be reproduced, stored in a retrieval system or transmitted in any form or by any means: electronic, electrostatic, magnetic, tape, mechanical photocopying, recording or otherwise without the written permission of the Publisher.

For permission to use material from this book please contact us:
Telephone 631-231-7269; Fax 631-231-8175
Web Site: http://www.novapublishers.com

### NOTICE TO THE READER

The Publisher has taken reasonable care in the preparation of this book, but makes no expressed or implied warranty of any kind and assumes no responsibility for any errors or omissions. No liability is assumed for incidental or consequential damages in connection with or arising out of information contained in this book. The Publisher shall not be liable for any special, consequential, or exemplary damages resulting, in whole or in part, from the readers' use of, or reliance upon, this material. Any parts of this book based on government reports are so indicated and copyright is claimed for those parts to the extent applicable to compilations of such works.

Independent verification should be sought for any data, advice or recommendations contained in this book. In addition, no responsibility is assumed by the publisher for any injury and/or damage to persons or property arising from any methods, products, instructions, ideas or otherwise contained in this publication.

This publication is designed to provide accurate and authoritative information with regard to the subject matter covered herein. It is sold with the clear understanding that the Publisher is not engaged in rendering legal or any other professional services. If legal or any other expert assistance is required, the services of a competent person should be sought. FROM A DECLARATION OF PARTICIPANTS JOINTLY ADOPTED BY A COMMITTEE OF THE AMERICAN BAR ASSOCIATION AND A COMMITTEE OF PUBLISHERS.

Additional color graphics may be available in the e-book version of this book.

**Library of Congress Cataloging-in-Publication Data**

ISBN: 978-1-63321-964-9

*Published by Nova Science Publishers, Inc. † New York*

# CONTENTS

**Preface** vii

**Chapter 1** Better Health Care and Lower Costs:
Accelerating Improvement through
Systems Engineering 1
*President's Council of Advisors
on Science and Technology*

**Chapter 2** Research Agenda for Healthcare
Systems Engineering 65
*Ronald L. Rardin*

**Index** 101

# PREFACE

Chapter 1 – This report identifies a comprehensive set of actions for enhancing health care across the Nation through greater use of systems-engineering principles. Systems engineering, widely used in manufacturing and aviation, is an interdisciplinary approach to analyze, design, manage, and measure a complex system in order to improve its efficiency, reliability, productivity, quality, and safety. It has often produced dramatically positive results in the small number of health-care organizations that have incorporated it into their processes. The report proposes a strategy that involves: (1) reforming payment systems, (2) building the Nation's health-data infrastructure, (3) providing technical assistance to providers, (4) increasing community collaboration, (5) sharing best practices, and (6) training health professionals in systems engineering approaches.

Chapter 2 – This report serves two primary functions: it (1) proposes a research agenda for health care systems engineering and (2) documents the funding challenges and potential funding solutions for health systems engineering. In this report, the health care system is conceptualized as consisting of six levels: patient, population, team, organization, network, and environment. The field of health care systems engineering is conceptualized as consisting of three domains: technology, model-based, and practice-based. A research agenda is outlined at each health care system level and the potential for advances is evaluated for each of the three health care systems engineering domains. Top research priorities identified include treatment optimization, personalized, preventive care, information rich and configurable operations management, collaboration within networks, and large-scale delivery system design.

In: A Systems Engineering Approach ...
Editor: Adeline Peaterson

ISBN: 978-1-63321-964-9
© 2014 Nova Science Publishers, Inc.

*Chapter 1*

# BETTER HEALTH CARE AND LOWER COSTS: ACCELERATING IMPROVEMENT THROUGH SYSTEMS ENGINEERING[*]

## President's Council of Advisors on Science and Technology

### EXECUTIVE SUMMARY

In recent years there has been success in expanding access to the health-care system, with millions gaining coverage in the past year due to the Affordable Care Act. With greater access, emphasis now turns to guaranteeing that care is both affordable and high-quality. Rising health-care costs are an important determinant of the Nation's fiscal future, and they also affect the budgets for States, businesses, and families across the country. Health-care costs now approach a fifth of the economy, and careful reviews suggest that a significant portion of those costs does not lead to better health or better care.

Other industries have used a range of systems-engineering approaches to reduce waste and increase reliability, and health care could benefit from adopting some of these approaches. As in those other industries, systems engineering has often produced dramatically positive results in the small number of health-care organizations that have implemented such concepts.

---

[*] This is an edited, reformatted and augmented version of a report to the President issued by the Office of Science and Technology Policy, May 2014.

These efforts have transformed health care at a small scale, such as improving the efficiency of a hospital pharmacy, and at much larger scales, such as coordinating operations across an entire hospital system or across a community. Systems tools and methods, moreover, can be used to ensure that care is reliably safe, to eliminate inefficient processes that do not improve care quality or people's health, and to ensure that health care is centered on patients and their families. Notwithstanding the instances in which these methods and techniques have been applied successfully, they remain underutilized throughout the broader system.

The primary barrier to greater use of systems methods and tools is the predominant fee-for-service payment system, which is a major disincentive to more efficient care. That system rewards procedures, not personalized care. To support needed change, the Nation needs to move more quickly to payment models that pay for value rather than volume. These new payment models depend on metrics to identify high-value care, which means that strong quality measures are needed, especially about health outcomes. With payment incentives aligned and quality information available, health care can take advantage of an array of approaches using systems engineering to redesign processes of care around the patient and bring community resources, as well as medical resources, together in support of that goal.

Additional barriers limit the spread and dissemination of systems methods and tools, such as insufficient data infrastructure and limited technical capabilities. These barriers are especially acute for practices with only one or a few physicians (small practices) or for community-wide efforts. To address these barriers, PCAST proposes the following overarching approaches where the Administration could make a difference:

1. Accelerate alignment of payment systems with desired outcomes,
2. Increase access to relevant health data and analytics,
3. Provide technical assistance in systems-engineering approaches,
4. Involve communities in improving health-care delivery,
5. Share lessons learned from successful improvement efforts, and
6. Train health professionals in new skills and approaches.

Through implementation of these strategies, systems tools and methods can play a major role in improving the value of the health-care system and improving the health of all Americans.

## SUMMARY OF RECOMMENDATIONS

**Recommendation 1**: Accelerate the alignment of payment incentives and reported information with better outcomes for individuals and populations.

> 1.1. Health and Human Services (HHS) should convene public and private payers (including Medicare, Medicaid, State programs, and commercial insurers) and employers to discuss how to accelerate the transition to outcomes-based payment, promote transparency, and provide tools and supports for practice transformation. This work could build on current alignment and measurement-improvement efforts at the Center for Medicare and Medicaid Services (CMS) and HHS broadly.
>
> 1.2. CMS should collaborate with the Agency for Healthcare Research and Quality (AHRQ) to develop the best measures (including outcomes) for patients and populations that can be readily assessed using current and future digital data sources. Such measures would create more meaningful information for providers and patients.

**Recommendation 2**: Accelerate efforts to develop the Nation's health-data infrastructure.

> 2.1. HHS should continue, and accelerate, the creation of a robust health-data infrastructure through widespread adoption of interoperable electronic health records and accessible health information. Specific actions in this vein were proposed in the 2010 PCAST report on health information technology and the related 2014 JASON report to the Office of the National Coordinator for Health Information Technology (ONC).

**Recommendation 3**: Provide national leadership in systems engineering by increasing the supply of data available to benchmark performance, understand a community's health, and examine broader regional or national trends.

3.1. HHS should create a senior leadership position, at the Assistant Secretary level, focused on health-care transformation to advance information science and data analytics. The duties for this position should include:
- Inventory existing data sources, identify opportunities for alignment and integration, and increase awareness of their potential;
- Expand access to existing data through open data initiatives;
- Promote collaboration with other Federal partners and private organizations; and
- Create a more focused and deep data-science capability through advancing data analytics and implementation of systems engineering.

3.2. HHS should work with the private sector to accelerate public- and private-payer release of provider-level data about quality, safety, and cost to increase transparency and enable patients to make more informed decisions.

**Recommendation 4**: Increase technical assistance (for a defined period—3-5 years) to health-care professionals and communities in applying systems approaches.

4.1. HHS should launch a large-scale initiative to provide hands-on support to small practices to develop the capabilities, skills, and tools to provide better, more coordinated care to their patients. This initiative should build on existing initiatives, such as the ONC Regional Extension Centers and the Department of Commerce's Manufacturing Extension Partnership.

**Recommendation 5**: Support efforts to engage communities in systematic health-care improvement.

5.1. HHS should continue to support State and local efforts to transform health care systems to provide better care quality and overall value.
5.2. Future CMS Innovation Center programs should, as appropriate, incorporate systems-engineering principles at the community level; set, assess, and achieve population-level goals; and encourage grantees to engage stakeholders outside of the traditional health-care system.

5.3. HHS should leverage existing community needs assessment and planning processes, such as the community health-needs assessments for non-profit hospitals, Accountable Care Organization (ACO) standards, health-department accreditation, and community health-center needs assessments, to promote systems thinking at the community level.

**Recommendation 6**: Establish awards, challenges, and prizes to promote the use of systems methods and tools in health care.

6.1. HHS and the Department of Commerce should build on the Baldrige awards to recognize health-care providers successfully applying system engineering approaches.

**Recommendation 7**: Build competencies and workforce for redesigning health care.

7.1. HHS should use a wide range of funding, program, and partnership levers to educate clinicians about systems-engineering competencies for scalable health-care improvement.
7.2. HHS should collect, inventory, and disseminate best practices in curricular and learning activities, as well as encourage knowledge sharing through regional learning communities. These functions could be accomplished through the new extension-center functions.
7.3. HHS should create grant programs for developing innovative health professional curricula that include systems engineering and implementation science, and HHS should disseminate the grant products broadly.
7.4. HHS should fund systems-engineering centers of excellence to build a robust specialty in Health- Improvement Science for physicians, nurses, health professionals, and administrators.

# INTRODUCTION AND MOTIVATION FOR IMPROVEMENT

In recent years, there has been success in expanding access to the health-care system, with millions gaining coverage in the past year due to the Affordable Care Act.[1] More than 8 million Americans signed up for health insurance between October 2013 and April 2014, and millions more gained coverage through Medicaid or their parents' health plan. With greater access, emphasis now turns to guaranteeing that care remains high-quality and is affordable. Rising health-care costs are affecting the Nation's fiscal future, and they also affect the budgets for States, businesses, and families across the country. Health-care costs now approach one-fifth of the economy, and careful reviews suggest that a significant portion of those costs does not lead to better health or better quality care.[2]

In addition to ensuring that care remains affordable, there is a need to center health care on patients, families, and population health. That objective requires action on multiple fronts, as stated well by the Institute of Medicine[3]: care should be safe, timely, effective, efficient, feasible and patient centered. There are opportunities to improve in each of these areas. For example, recent reviews suggest that over one-quarter of Medicare patients experienced some type of harm during a hospital stay, and other research finds that between one-fifth to one- third of all hospitalized patients experienced a medical error. Almost half of these errors were likely preventable.[4] Other studies suggest that patients are not routinely involved in decisions about their treatments or managing their conditions. And anecdotal evidence and studies highlight the impact inefficiencies have on patients—long waits for appointments, information not transmitted between clinicians, and patients with complex diseases feeling lost trying to get the care they need.

These shortfalls are occurring even as most clinicians work tirelessly for their patients. Their work is frustrated by processes that contain unnecessary burdens and inefficiencies, with some studies suggesting that almost one- third of front-line health-care workers' time is wasted.[5] The current stresses on clinicians mean that improvement initiatives cannot simply add to a clinician's workload or rely on the clinicians finding time to participate in additional initiatives. Rather, successful and sustainable improvement must involve reconfiguring the workflow and overall environment in which these professionals practice, which can help to reduce the burden of work while improving the performance of the system.

Making such changes in an integrated manner is the essence of systems engineering. Recent policies, deriving from the Affordable Care Act and the American Recovery and Reinvestment Act,[6] have laid the groundwork for wider use of systems engineering through new care models that promote integrated care and rapid adoption of electronic health records. The National Quality Strategy identifies areas for improvement in health-care quality and outcomes that systems-engineering initiatives need to address.[7] The current policy environment and advances in technical capabilities combine to make this the right time to focus on expanding systems methods and tools throughout health care.

## SUCCESSFUL USE OF SYSTEMS ENGINEERING IN OTHER INDUSTRIES

Other industries have used a range of approaches, known collectively as systems engineering, to improve productivity, efficiency, reliability, and quality. For example, by using tools such as alerts, redundancies, checklists, and systems that adjust for the human factor,[8] U.S. commercial airlines have reduced fatalities from hundreds in the 1960s to approaching zero now, with the risk of dying from flying now at 1 in 45 million flights. They have also been used in fields as diverse as manufacturing, space stations and satellites, and education.

Systems tools and methods draw on many fields of expertise, including multiple types of engineering, scientific fields, social sciences, and management, as well as the circumstances of different industries. Given the diversity of fields involved, multiple terms are used to describe this concept. For the purposes of this report, we use the term systems engineering to include the full suite of tools and methods that can analyze a system, its elements, and connections between elements; assist with the design of policies and processes; and help manage operations to provide better quality and outcomes at lower cost (see Box 1 and the appendices for further information on systems engineering, including definitions of key terms).[9]

## PROMISE OF SYSTEMS ENGINEERING FOR HEALTH AND HEALTH CARE

Health care could benefit from the range of available systems-engineering approaches. In the small number of health-care organizations that have implemented these concepts, systems engineering has often produced dramatically positive results. Systems engineering can help reengineer critical-care environments to improve both the patient experience and the effectiveness of care, such as coordinating the different devices monitoring the patient's health, reducing false alarms that prevent the patient from resting, and connecting monitors to therapeutic equipment so that action can be taken immediately when a problem is identified.[10] There are successful examples at different scales, ranging from improving the efficiency of a single hospital pharmacy to coordinating operations across an entire hospital system or across a community. Table 1 illustrates the diversity of tools and methods that could be used for different settings or segments of the health-care system, along with the challenges that these approaches could help address, and Box 2 provides an example on taking a systems approach to improve care across a community.

---

### BOX 1. OVERVIEW OF SYSTEMS ENGINEERING

*What is it?* An interdisciplinary approach to analyze, design, manage, and measure a complex system with efforts to improve its efficiency, productivity, quality, safety, and other factors. For the purposes of this report, the term systems engineering includes the full suite of tools and methods that can analyze a system, its elements, and connections between elements; assist with the design of policies and processes; and help manage operations to provide better quality and outcomes at lower cost.

*How can it be applied?* Systems-engineering processes can be applied in multiple ways depending on the specific challenges and the type of system, with the model below highlighting the types of steps taken. Systems engineering is most successful when data are harnessed at each stage in the cycle.

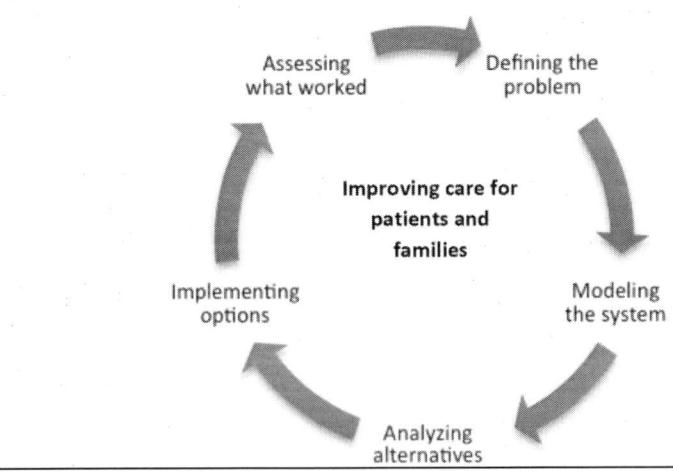

---

> ***What types of systems methods and tools are used now?*** Multiple strategies are available, although their usefulness depends on the specific type of health care. Some examples include:
>
> - industrial engineering
> - production-system methods, Lean, and broader process-improvement techniques
> - operations management, queuing theory, and patient-flow variability
> - high-reliability approaches
> - human-factors engineering
> - complexity science
> - statistical process control
> - modeling and simulation
> - supply-chain management
> - systematic management techniques (e.g., total-quality management)
> - safety tools (e.g., root-cause analysis, checklists, health-care failure modes and effect analyses)

Denver Health, a health system that serves the most vulnerable, safety-net populations in Colorado, is an excellent example of how an organization used the Toyota Production System to redesign its entire operations. It started by mapping out its operations and found significant waste, with one industrial engineer finding that its trauma- surgery resident physicians walked 8 ½ miles during a 24-hour shift. It sought to reduce this waste using Lean techniques, rapidly testing new ideas to improve a high-priority problem. The Lean techniques have helped the organization achieve specific successes—such as reducing two serious conditions (deep-vein thrombosis and pulmonary embolism) by 80 percent and by halving the time needed to prepare a hospital room for the next patient. On a broader scale, Denver Health has saved almost $200 million since it began its work in 2006 and reduced its mortality rate to some of the lowest among its peers in academic health centers.[11] It has achieved these successes while seeing a 60 percent increase in uncompensated care, illustrating the wide range of organizations that could take advantage of these approaches.[12]

**Table 1. Potential impact of systems engineering on different segments of the health system, showing selected challenges alongside potential systems methods and tools approaches**

| Health system stakeholder | Selected challenges | Example systems methods and tools to address selected challenges |
|---|---|---|
| *Patients* | • Uncoordinated care<br>• Inefficient use of their time and effort<br>• Care not centered on their needs, goals, and circumstances | • Operations management to ensure resources are available when needed<br>• Checklists or dashboards to ensure reliable care delivery<br>• Reengineering processes to incorporate patient input |
| *Small clinical practices* | • Clinician stress and burnout<br>• Inefficient workflows for delivering care<br>• Inconsistent usability of different health-information tools<br>• Uneven delivery of evidence-based prevention and treatment | • Lean techniques for eliminating waste in workflows and clinical processes<br>• Human-factors engineering techniques to ensure health-information tools are easily usable |
| *Large health-care organizations* | • Managing new payment models that reward outcomes vs. process<br>• Errors and gaps in care<br>• Wasted resources from inefficient workflows<br>• Wasted resources from unnecessary administrative processes | • Standardized protocols that incorporate new evidence and can be tailored to individual patients<br>• Predictive analytics to identify potential risks before problems occur<br>• Supply-chain management to minimize waste in supplies and pharmaceuticals |
| *Communities* | • Little coordination among community organizations, local governments, and health-care organizations<br>• Partnering to address the many factors that affect people's health | • Modeling how policies can build on community resources<br>• Operations research to identify at-risk community members and efficiently deliver preventive health services<br>• Big-data methods for identifying patients who need more intensive coordination of their health care |

Another strong example is Kaiser Permanente, one of the Nation's largest managed-care organizations. Kaiser uses multiple approaches, including systems engineering, to continually update the way it delivers care and to ensure that new scientific evidence is consistently applied. These tools for performance improvement include a web- based data dashboard that tracks performance across medical centers and geographic areas, corps of improvement advisors, enhanced clinical-information systems, staff training in performance improvement, and systems for sharing technical knowledge.[13] While these tools have been applied to multiple aspects of care, one illustrative example was their application to improving care for sepsis, a potentially fatal condition brought on by severe infection. This condition is serious as it is often only detected when it is too late to help the patient. After identifying sepsis as an opportunity for improvement, two hospitals began rapid-cycle pilot testing of approaches to detect and treat this difficult condition quickly. The broader organization spread the technical and cultural interventions that were needed to implement this work successfully in other hospitals. As a result of this new approach, Kaiser was able to identify three times as many sepsis cases, treat those patients quickly, and cut mortality from this condition by half.[14]

> While there are excellent examples, systems methods and tools are still not used on a widespread basis through health care.

Unfortunately, these examples are rare in U.S. health care. Many organizations and communities that could benefit from these tools and methods are not applying them to their operations.

---

### Box 2. Taking a Systems Approach to Improve Care across a Community[15]

Seeking to improve the health of Americans across a large region of Tennessee and Kentucky, Vanderbilt University Medical Center and its affiliates confronted the question of how to scale up a program they knew worked for people with chronic disease.[16] Their challenge was how to help patients across a broad community improve their control of chronic conditions—such as high blood pressure, heart disease, and diabetes—and help coordinate the care for patients discharged from the hospital for serious conditions— such as heart attacks or pneumonia.

By improving people's health, the program could help people stay healthy at home, which would also reduce the overall cost of care, instead of having to return to the hospital or go to the emergency room.

The initiative was built around a model for health-care delivery, called MyHealthTeam, where teams of primary care clinicians, specialists, and care coordinators work together to care for patients using health information technology. The project uses real-time dashboards to track how patients are doing and to ensure care is delivered reliably. The model identifies those in greatest need of health care, so that clinicians can focus their attention on those that need it most. Once identified, those patients at highest risk of health problems are connected with a clinician who rapidly applies evidence-based interventions to find what works for the patient.

This program is based on earlier initiatives that improved hypertension care by educating clinicians about best practices, providing regular feedback to clinicians, providing education tools for patients, and building on technologies that have been successfully used to coordinate clinical care. All of this relies on a significant data infrastructure that includes information about hospital discharges, labs, administrative data, data recorded by the patient, surveys, and Federal and State data. By integrating different data together, the program is able to identify patterns, understand outcomes, and support clinical decisions. MyHealthTeam also applies systems engineering through regular improvement cycles, streamlining inefficient workflows, employing health-care professionals strategically, and using technology.

The project has experienced several challenges in scaling the model to larger populations and additional clinical groups. These include different organizational cultures, trust, concerns about change, dealing with payment-model changes, staff bandwidth and time, and exchanging information across different information systems. To overcome these challenges, the initiative has developed several strategies, such as developing effective working relationships with community partners, providing technical support to assist with data challenges, and always considering efficiencies when asking partners to take on new work. During its expansion phase, MyHealthTeam is tracking 5 outcomes: disease control, reduce hospital admissions, reduce emergency room usage, reduce total cost of care, and reduce the cost per beneficiary per month. It has already seen improvements in the control of chronic diseases, and further work will be needed to understand the other outcomes.

# FACTORS LIMITING DISSEMINATION AND SPREAD OF SYSTEMS-ENGINEERING PRINCIPLES

Barriers to greater use of systems methods and tools include the lack of quality and performance measures and the misaligned incentive structure of the predominant fee-for-service payment system, which encourages a fragmented delivery system. To support needed change, the Nation needs to move more quickly to payment models that pay for value.[17] These approaches depend on metrics to identify high-value care, which means that strong quality measures are needed, especially about health outcomes. With payment incentives aligned and quality information available, health care can take advantage of an array of approaches using systems engineering to redesign the process of care around the patient and bring community resources, as well as medical resources, together in support of that goal.

Another challenge is an organization's leadership and culture, which determine people's commitment to improvement efforts.[18] For example, one systems-engineering initiative achieved some success by using checklists to reduce infections among severely ill patients, but significant improvement did not occur until there was a culture where everyone felt they were able to speak up about potential safety concerns.[19] Other barriers include technical challenges, workforce capabilities, and limited knowledge about what works.

The siloed nature of the health system, in which clinical care is separated in an uncoordinated fashion across multiple specialties and settings, presents another challenge that can limit the use of systems approaches. Clinicians often focus only on the activities in their particular silo, as opposed to considering the broader concerns of the patient. Moving away from the current siloed state requires systematic knowledge of the many processes and providers involved in a given patient's care, as well as a cultural shift toward team-based care where all work together to address a patient's needs.

There are additional challenges for clinicians working in small practices. Small practices provide a significant number of Americans with their care—despite trends toward consolidation, as of 2012 nearly 60 percent of physicians were still in practices with 10 or fewer physicians (see Figure 1).[20] The distribution of clinicians is changing rapidly, and there has been a significant increase in the fraction of physician practices owned by hospitals in the last several years. Data are continuing to emerge on the extent of this affiliation and consolidation trend.[21]

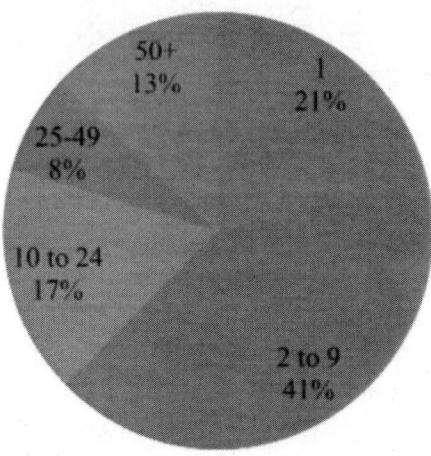

Figure 1. Distribution of Physicians by Practice Size, 2012.[22]

The physicians, nurses, and other personnel in small practices often are juggling many responsibilities to keep the practice operating, have fewer resources to invest in technical infrastructure or new improvement methods, and may not have the resources to hire staff specifically dedicated to implementing systems-engineering techniques. As a result, the clinicians in these practices often have to squeeze any improvement efforts in between seeing patients, documenting their clinical evaluations, coordinating care, and handling administrative paperwork for billing and reimbursement.

Given these barriers, successful spread of systems engineering will depend on multiple strategies that account for the diversity of American health care.[23] PCAST proposes the following overarching goals where the Administration could make a difference in the adoption of these methods and tools:

1. Accelerate alignment of payment systems with desired outcomes,
2. Increase access to relevant health data and analytics,
3. Provide technical assistance in systems-engineering approaches,
4. Involve communities in improving health-care delivery
5. Share lessons learned from successful improvement efforts, and
6. Train health professionals in new skills and approaches.

These recommendations together form a systems approach, with the potential for positive interactions among them. Since progress will depend on collaborations among providers, communities, and others, all recommendations in this report should be viewed through that lens. This report discusses these areas in more detail and provides detailed recommendations to accelerate adoption of systems-engineering approaches across the Nation.

## GOAL 1. ACCELERATE ALIGNMENT OF PAYMENT SYSTEMS WITH DESIRED OUTCOMES

The current payment system is a major barrier to progress. The predominant way clinicians and hospitals are paid for health care discourages real improvement as it rewards higher volumes of tests and treatments over whether a patient has a better outcome. At the same time, clinicians are not paid for activities that are known to improve a patient's health—such as coordinating a patient's care or talking with a patient about whether a treatment meets his or her needs. Perhaps most irrationally, a hospital is paid more when patients have complications, so that preventing patient harm can actually cause revenues to decline.[24] As the current incentive system limits improvement broadly, systems engineering is not immune from its effects (see Box 3 for one example).

---

**BOX 3. VIRGINIA MASON MEDICAL CENTER BACK PAIN CLINIC EXAMPLE — HOW PAYMENT POLICIES CAN DISCOURAGE SYSTEMS ENGINEERING**[25]

While changing the payment system for health care is important for many reasons, it has specific importance for the use of systems methods and tools. One example of this occurred for Virginia Mason Medical Center in Seattle, Washington, which uses the Toyota Production System to optimize its operations. As a result of its use of that system, the organization has some of the lowest rates of serious hospital complications, such as infections and falls; has reduced its medical-malpractice liability by almost 40 percent; and has been recognized as one of the top hospitals in the country in both quality and efficiency. When Virginia Mason redesigned its back-pain clinic, it reduced patient waiting times, reduced the use of unnecessary tests, lowered costs, and got people back to work and their desired function. In spite of these positive impacts, revenues decreased because Virginia Mason reduced the use of expensive services, such as MRIs, and increased the use of lower-cost services such as physical therapy.

> It was initially able to keep the program operational by negotiating with local employers to change how they paid for back care, while working on other operational improvements to continue this service lines profitability. This specific experience highlights the unintended consequences that can occur under the current payment system, as well as the importance of engaging more elements from the community in which health care is delivered.

To address the perverse incentives now in place, the Affordable Care Act (ACA) included multiple programs that move toward payment that rewards better health outcomes at lower cost. For example, 360 accountable care organizations (ACOs) are now providing care to more than 5 million Medicare beneficiaries,[26] and hundreds more ACOs are operating for commercially insured patients. Yet this transition is not complete, as providers may be operating under multiple payment programs at the same time—some focused on health outcomes and value, while others continue to pay solely on quantity of services. As a result, a provider can be rewarded by some programs for improving their patients' health, while losing money from other programs because those patients are using fewer health-care services.[27] In order to overcome this problem, the Administration should work with the private sector to accelerate the transition of the payment system so that clinicians receive consistent incentives across all public and private health-insurance plans to deliver high-quality and high-value health care.[28]

New payment models will require performance measures that assess health outcomes, not just the process of care, which is the primary focus of current metrics. Transitioning performance metrics from processes to patient outcomes will allow benchmarking between systems and providers. Better measurement science can lay the foundation for more effective measures for public and private accountability programs, while eliminating metrics with weak impact on quality or risk of unintended consequences. It will be critical to develop outcomes-based measures and align these "measures that matter" across payers, as the current proliferation of measures frustrates providers and requires significant resources to collect, store, and report.[29]

In addition to payment, measurement can help drive improvement by increasing the amount of information available for clinicians, health-care organizations, and patients. Improving the measures available will ensure that initiatives using systems methods and tools will focus their effort on what matters. In some cases, the data may not be available, while in others the challenge is turning existing data into meaningful information.

**Recommendation 1**: Accelerate the alignment of payment incentives and reported information with better outcomes for individuals and broader populations.

 1.1. Health and Human Services (HHS) should convene public and private payers (including Medicare, Medicaid, State programs, and commercial insurers) and employers to discuss how to accelerate the transition to outcomes-based payments, promote transparency, and provide tools and supports for practice transformation. This work could build on current alignment and measurement improvement efforts at the Center for Medicare and Medicaid Services (CMS) and HHS broadly.

 1.2. CMS should collaborate with the Agency for Healthcare Research and Quality (AHRQ) to develop the best measures (including outcomes) for patients and populations that can be readily assessed using current and future digital data sources. Such measures would create more meaningful information for providers and for patients.

## GOAL 2. INCREASE ACCESS TO RELEVANT HEALTH DATA AND ANALYTICS

Systems engineering requires multiple types of data to be successful, ranging from clinical health information to information on operational processes to broader benchmarking indicators. As data sets approach the size that can be deemed "big data," new capabilities emerge that can assist system-improvement efforts. From understanding what treatments work to conveying the multiple factors (system, provider, and environmental) that contribute to health outcomes, big data bears the potential to support predictive medicine--clinicians may anticipate who will develop disease or predict what treatments will be successful for a given patient. While some of the needed data are currently collected and available, greater work is needed to expand the data sets required to reach these capabilities.

## Expanding Clinical and Operational Data for Improvement Initiatives

The amount of electronic clinical data available to clinicians and healthcare organizations has been increasing due to the HITECH Act[30] and associated incentives from Medicare and Medicaid for providers to adopt and use electronic health records (EHRs). EHRs are a vital tool to support data-driven systems engineering approaches in health care, yet many organizations still lack a comprehensive EHR system, and others are still learning how to use these digital tools to improve care. These problems are especially acute in smaller practices that may lack the infrastructure that larger organizations possess. Providers need hands-on support to develop the expertise and business processes to improve care using health information technology (IT).

Greater amounts of data are not helpful if they are not of good quality and easily exchangeable among all of the clinicians involved in a patient's care. Good quality data are accurate, complete, timely, relevant, and consistent; adherence to standards for data quality would ensure the reliability of both data and analytics. Interoperability among EHR systems remains a challenge, and future progress will depend on interoperability among a wide range of digital and mobile data sources. The Office of the National Coordinator for Health Information Technology (ONC) has focused on expanding interoperability, and CMS and ONC have included interoperability as a key requirement for the "meaningful-use" incentive program. Further efforts in these programs will address this challenge.

Another source of data for improving care is patient-generated health data.[31] Incorporating data generated directly by the patient, which is largely unharnessed by the health system today, presents the opportunity not only to improve clinical care and patient engagement, but also gives researchers a more comprehensive view of the patient experience. Given the expected surge of such data in coming years, the Federal Government may be able to help make the data more accessible to patients and clinicians by developing standards and providing incentives for utilizing and integrating this information.[32] Some action is already under way—ONC's Federal advisory committees are exploring ways to add patient-generated data into Meaningful Use Stage 3 guidelines,[33] while the National Institutes of Health (NIH) supports the Patient Reported Outcomes Measurement Information System to provide reliable and precise measures of patient-reported health status.

Beyond clinical information, many systems-engineering approaches require data on operational processes, from the flow of patients through different units of a hospital to the time it takes clinicians to complete specific tasks. When collected, these data are often in different systems than clinical information, and they may not be collected in a format that can be easily applied to system redesign. Smaller practices may be especially challenged to routinely collect this type of data and have data systems that can store them.

There are several policy options to continue and accelerate the development of a robust health IT infrastructure, such as those described in the 2010 PCAST Health IT report and the 2014 JASON report for ONC (see Box 4 and the appendices for further information).[34] These analyses continue to be relevant as future Federal health IT policies are developed.

**Recommendation 2**: Accelerate efforts to develop the Nation's health data infrastructure.

2.1. Health and Human Services should continue, and accelerate, the creation of a robust health-data infrastructure through widespread adoption of interoperable electronic health records and advances in data exchange. Specific actions in this vein were proposed in the 2010 PCAST report on health information technology and the related 2014 JASON report to the Office of the National Coordinator for Health Information Technology.

## Expanding Data Available for Assessing Progress

While local clinical and operational data sources are critical, additional data are needed to benchmark performance, understand a community's health, and examine broader regional or national trends. These data are critical for successful systems reengineering, as they can help an organization or community identify opportunities for improvement and assess their progress in real time. Data already collected by HHS could be leveraged to serve many of these purposes, as illustrated in Table 2, and could help foster partnerships that translate these resources into meaningful information for improvement.

> **BOX 4. KEY CONCLUSIONS FROM 2010 PCAST REPORT AND 2014 JASON REPORT ON HEALTH IT**
>
> 1. HHS's vigorous efforts have laid a foundation for progress in the adoption of health IT, with historic increases in the use of electronic health records by clinicians in the last several years.
> 2. Data interoperability across EHR systems remains a substantial barrier to the development of a robust health IT infrastructure to support new care models and to health information exchange among providers and with patients to support patient care.
> 3. Both reports called on HHS to advance standards and services to make it easier to pull data from EHRs and exchange it, as well as to build these requirements into meaningful use guidelines. Each report had the same goal, but recommended slightly different technical solutions for achieving the vision:
>    a. The 2010 PCAST report called for the development of a "universal exchange language" that enables health IT data to be shared across institutions and the creation of the infrastructure that permits physicians and patients to combine patient data across institutional boundaries.
>    b. By contrast, the 2014 JASON report recommended that EHR vendors be required to develop and publish APIs for medical-records data and demonstrate that data from their EHRs can be exchanged via these APIs and used in a meaningful way by third-party software developers.
>
> EHR interoperability is not merely a feat of technology. Once accomplished, it can help to make more data available for the kinds of analyses that enable systems engineering. It can also help practices (of any size) that have adopted EHRs serve their patients better because it will be easier for them to draw on and use data from the multiple sources where patients have received care.

HHS has already started sharing these data more broadly though its open-data initiative, which is part of its broader open-government plan. Many of these data are now posted on HealthData.gov, which has catalogued over 1,000 HHS data sets along with data sets from multiple states.[35] In addition, the Centers for Medicare and Medicaid Services (CMS) established the Office of Information Products and Data Analytics to maximize the use of CMS data by internal and external users (see Box 5).

**Table 2. Example data resources throughout the Department of Health and Human Services**

| Selected HHS agencies and offices | Selected data resources |
|---|---|
| **Administration for Children & Families** | Child Welfare Outcomes data, Head Start and Early Head Start program statistics |
| **Administration for Community Living** | National Residential Information Systems Project, National Survey of Area Agencies on Aging, National Survey of Older Americans Act Participants |
| **Agency for Healthcare Research and Quality** | National Healthcare Quality Report, National Healthcare Disparities Report, State Snapshots, Healthcare Cost and Utilization Project; Medical Expenditure Panel Survey [collaboration with CDC and Census Bureau], National Quality Measures Clearinghouse |
| **Agency for Toxic Substances & Disease Registry** | National Amyotrophic Lateral Sclerosis (ALS)Registry, National Toxic Substance Incidents Program, Rapid Response Registry survey instrument, Toxicological profiles for hazardous substances |
| **Centers for Disease Control and Prevention** | National Center for Health Statistics, National Vital Statistics System, National Health Interview Survey, National Health and Nutrition Examination Survey, National Health Care Surveys, Behavioral Risk Factor Surveillance System, National Program of Cancer Registries, Health Indicators Warehouse, WONDER online databases |
| **Centers for Medicare & Medicaid Services** | Hospital Compare, Physician Compare, Office of Information Products and Data Analytics, Hospital Charge Data, Nursing Home Compare, Physician Charge Data, National Health Expenditure Data, Medicaid Statistical Information System, Medicare Current Beneficiary Survey, Chronic Conditions Data Warehouse, Medicare claims data, Medicaid Statistical Information System data |
| **Food and Drug Administration** | Adverse Event Reporting System, Premarket Approvals, Recalls Database |

## Table 2. (Continued)

| Selected HHS agencies and offices | Selected data resources |
|---|---|
| **Health Resources and Services Administration** | Uniform Data System for health centers, Health Resources Comparison Tool, Health Professional Shortage Areas, National Center for Health Workforce Analysis data |
| **Office of the National Coordinator for Health IT** | Health IT Dashboard, National Survey on Health Information Exchange in Clinical Laboratories, Regional Extension Center program activity |
| **National Institutes of Health** | Health Information National Trends Survey; Patient Reported Outcomes Measurement Information System [PROMIS]; Surveillance, Epidemiology, and End Results Program [SEER] |
| **Substance Abuse & Mental Health Services Administration** | National Registry of Evidence-based Programs and Practices, National Survey on Drug Use and Health, Drug Abuse Warning Network, Behavioral Health Services Information System, Treatment Episode Data Set |

One example of the transformative impact of open data in another industry is the Energy Information Administration (EIA), which serves as an objective and independent source of energy information on a wide range of issues—imports and exports, supply and demand, and production and inventories—for different energy sources; analyzes the source data to produce actionable information; and disseminates that information broadly. The legislation that created the EIA ensured that its products are released directly without a clearance process from other Department of Energy (DOE) offices, the Secretary, or the Office of Management and Budget (OMB), which has been important for its independence and objectivity. As a result, its products serve as a definitive source of energy information for the Federal government, private sector, and the public; help to inform policy; help businesses understand the energy landscape; and help the public see broader trends and challenges.[38]

There are also additional health data sources beyond HHS that could be leveraged—including other Federal sources, such as the Federal Employee Health Benefit Program, Veterans Health Administration (VHA), and the

Department of Defense (DoD). Public-private partnerships that produce publicly available reports, such as the Patient-Centered Outcomes Research Institute (PCORI), also serve as useful data sources. PCORI conducts comparative effectiveness and patient-centered outcomes research. Disseminating comparative-effectiveness research and related scientific information to providers at the point of care enables improvement of clinical processes and provides an evidence base for improvement initiatives centered on better health at lower cost.

> **BOX 5. CMS IS MAKING MEDICARE CLAIMS DATA AVAILABLE TO ENROLLEES, RESEARCHERS, ACCOUNTABLE CARE ORGANIZATIONS, QUALITY REPORTING ORGANIZATIONS, AND THE PUBLIC[36]**
>
> - Researchers can now access Medicare claims data through CMS' Virtual Research Data Center (VRDC), a secure and efficient means for researchers to virtually access and analyze CMS's vast store of health care data, at a much lower cost than traditional data-access mechanisms.
> - CMS is providing Accountable Care Organizations (ACOs) with monthly claims feeds covering the almost 3 million beneficiaries being cared for by physicians participating in the ACOs.
> - To help States coordinate care, CMS is now providing over 30 States with timely Medicare data for dual-eligible beneficiaries. Medicare data are an essential tool for States as they try to improve quality and control costs for these beneficiaries.
> - The ACA authorized CMS to share Medicare data with approved qualified entities (QEs) for the purposes of provider quality reporting. QEs combine Medicare claims data from CMS with claims data from other payers to create comprehensive reports on the performance of hospitals, physicians, and other health-care providers.
> - Beginning three years ago, Medicare enrollees have access to their own claims information.[37]
> - CMS is publicly releasing Medicare data at the provider level to promote transparency and spur innovation.

- In May 2013, CMS released detailed information on average hospital charges for the 100 most common Medicare in-patient admissions, followed in June by data on selected out- patient procedures. These data have been downloaded more than 260,000 times, sparking a national debate on observed variation in hospital charges.
- In April 2014 CMS released detailed information on services and procedures provided to Medicare beneficiaries by physicians and other health-care professionals. These data included more than 9 million lines of information, collectively covering more than 880,000 unique providers, and provided unprecedented insights into how care is delivered in the Medicare program. Within the first week of posting, more than 150,000 users downloaded these data, which can be used to help consumers and other stakeholders compare the services provided and payments received by individual health-care providers.

Given the multiple resources currently available—from the National Center for Health Statistics to National Healthcare Quality Reports to Medicare claims data—HHS does not need to create a centralized data office. Progress would be accelerated, however, by inventorying data from multiple sources (including Federal health and social-support programs, Federal surveys, and public-health and surveillance programs), and building HHS' capacity to analyze, use and release data across many sources. These rich data can help to reveal the multiple determinants of health, understand how a community's context may lead to specific health challenges, and evaluate different interventions and strategies to improve health. Technical work would be needed to make these data actionable, and additional data-security and privacy protections would be required before these are broadly distributed.

**Recommendation 3**: Provide national leadership in systems engineering by increasing the supply of data available to benchmark performance, understand a community's health, and examine broader regional or national trends.

3.1. Health and Human Services should create a senior leadership position, at the Assistant Secretary level, focused on health-care transformation. The duties for this position should include:

- Inventory existing data sources, identify opportunities for alignment and integration, and increase awareness of their potential;
- Expand access to existing data through open-data initiatives;
- Promote collaboration with other Federal partners and private organizations; and
- Create a more focused and deep data-science capability through advancing data analytics and implementation of systems engineering.

3.2. HHS should work with the private sector to accelerate public and private payer release of provider-level data about quality, safety, and cost to increase transparency and enable patients to make more informed decisions.

(See Appendix G for illustrative examples of ways to build HHS data-science leadership).

## GOAL 3. PROVIDE TECHNICAL ASSISTANCE IN SYSTEMS-ENGINEERING APPROACHES

Health-care professionals and administrators will need technical support to apply systems-engineering approaches throughout their operations. This is especially true for clinicians working in smaller practices, who tend to have fewer technical capabilities available. Similarly, there are challenges when communities seek to apply systems methods and tools to improving the health of their community, as they, too, may have limited tools at their disposal.

One of the earliest efforts to provide "boots-on-the-ground" support was through the agricultural Cooperative Extension System.[39] As described in recent publications,[40] the Extension System played a critical role in teaching farmers about new farming practices, developing new evidence on what worked, and helping people adapt the research to their particular situation. This concept has been successfully applied to other sectors of the economy, such as through the Hollings Manufacturing Extension Partnership (MEP) at the National Institute of Standards and Technology (NIST) within the Department of Commerce. The MEP consists of regional centers that provide technical, scientific, and managerial assistance to smaller American manufacturing companies to identify and adopt new technologies. Surveys of participating companies have found positive impacts, reporting that companies have had $2.5 billion in new sales, saved $900 million in their costs, and created or retained over 60,000 jobs.[41]

Efforts to expand technical assistance in systems engineering can build on several existing efforts. The Veterans Health Administration (VHA) established Veterans Engineering Research Centers in 2009 to develop innovative care delivery models, incorporate engineering principles into health care, create education and training programs to share knowledge between engineering and health-care fields and provide guidance on engineering principles more broadly. Another health-care technical assistance effort is through the Quality Improvement Organizations (QIOs) and Quality Innovation Networks (QINs) supported by the Centers for Medicare and Medicaid Services (CMS), which work directly with Medicare providers to improve the effectiveness, efficiency, and quality of Medicare services. Similarly, the CMS Innovation Center has funded a three-year project, led by the Northeastern University Healthcare Systems Engineering Institute, to test the impact and viability of a network of health-care systems-engineering regional extension centers. And the Agency for Healthcare Research and Quality (AHRQ) recently announced support for a network of centers to assist small and medium-sized primary-care practices in implementing patient-centered outcomes research findings and building the capacity in such practices for incorporating this evidence moving forward.[42]

Another example of the extension-service model is offered by the Regional Extension Centers (RECs) overseen by the Office of the National Coordinator for Health Information Technology (ONC), which seek to help providers with the adoption of electronic health records (EHRs) and health IT. These centers are particularly focused on providing technical support to clinicians in small, rural, and underserved areas and helping them become meaningful users of health IT. Several studies have suggested the RECs have been successful in supporting providers to achieve this goal. A Government Accountability Office study found that providers working with RECs were almost twice as likely to use EHR systems meaningfully compared to others.[43] Another recent study found that the RECs recruited over 130,000 primary-care providers, leading to 90 percent of these clinicians using an advanced EHR and almost half using health IT meaningfully.[44]

There is also an opportunity to foster partnerships among organizations that operate with a strong, corporate process structure–Six Sigma, Lean, total quality management (TQM), and others–with their local health care systems providing care to the very people who make up those organizations. This type of public-private partnership should be encouraged as it allows "localization and adaptation" of conventional systems engineering in health-care settings. It also creates an environment where the skills of high-performing companies, which have incorporated systems engineering into their processes, can be applied to teach, reengineer, and/or otherwise support a local hospital directly. It should in no way, however, be a substitute for what the market can and should develop, i.e., for-profit organizations that provide training and skills to health-care systems.

**Recommendation 4**: Increase technical assistance (for a defined period of 3-5 years) to health-care professionals and communities in applying systems approaches.

> 4.1. Health and Human Services should launch a large-scale initiative to provide hands-on support to small practices to develop the capabilities, skills, and tools to provide better, more coordinated care to their patients. This initiative should build on existing initiatives, such as the Office of the National Coordinator for Health Information Technology Regional Extension Centers and the Department of Commerce's Manufacturing Extension Partnership.

## GOAL 4. INVOLVE COMMUNITIES IN IMPROVING HEALTH-CARE DELIVERY

Currently, systems-engineering principles have mostly been applied within health-care organizations, as those organizations have technical capabilities and structures for implementing these methods and tools. Yet, not all clinicians practice in larger organizations, and people spend most of their lives outside of the traditional health- care system. A systems approach that optimizes the contributions of community resources and promotes coordination across various providers and agencies in a community will increase the likelihood of providing better health at lower cost.

### Positive Results Occur When Partnering with Communities

For example, health-care delivery can improve when reengineering brings together health care and community partners, often using the patient-centered medical home concept as a key element. The work of Jeffrey Brenner in Camden, New Jersey provides a positive example of how clinicians can partner with non-clinical teams to serve the needs of severely ill patients, thereby better managing their condition while saving money.[45] Technical assistance is needed to accomplish this type of reengineering at the community level, such as teaching communities how to review community data, identify opportunities based on maps of health status patterns, and consider potentially relevant evidence-based programs to address those issues. (See Box 6 for an example of community involvement in care).

> ### BOX 6. IMPROVING CARE TRANSITIONS WITH THE COMMUNITY—CARE NETWORK[47]
>
> Many patients return to the hospital shortly after being discharged—almost one-fifth of Medicare patients and one-tenth of privately insured adults return to the hospital within a month, although this rate has declined recently.[48] There are multiple reasons why it is a challenge to keep patients healthy when they leave the hospital, from helping patients understand their treatment, to ensuring medication and supplies are available, to arranging transportation to appointments, to accommodating patients' overall living conditions. Some of these challenges can be met directly by the health-care system, while others require partnerships with the community.
>
> Queen of the Valley Medical Center, in Napa County, California, developed an initiative to help patients stay healthy as they transitioned from the hospital to their home. The effort focused specifically on reducing readmissions to hospitals and emergency-room use for low-income adults and vulnerable older adults with complex health needs, using the CARE Network (Case Management, Advocacy, Resource/Referral, Education) for addressing these challenges. There are specific challenges for implementing this work in Napa County given the diversity of its population, number of languages spoken, and varying socioeconomic status (with one-quarter of the population living below 200 percent of the Federal poverty line).
>
> The CARE network uses a team-based approach to ensure that a patient's needs are being met, coordinating between medical services and other resources.

> For example, a team consisting of a social worker and nurse will visit the patient at home to ensure a patient knows how to manage his or her treatment and to discuss the supports needed to make that happen—housing, food, transportation to medical appointments, behavioral health needs, and necessary medications. In some cases, this may involve help in navigating the health-care system; in other cases this may involve coordinating with social services and community organizations. The team continues to visit the home until the patient has the knowledge and support services to manage his or her own care and health.
>
> Early results are promising. During the 2012 fiscal year, the program was associated with a 50 percent reduction in hospitalizations and a 60 percent decrease in using the emergency room, while the patients were 20 percent less likely to be readmitted to the hospital compared to similar patients.

System-based design can be helpful when rebuilding a community's health infrastructure after a crisis. Following Hurricane Katrina, the health-care infrastructure was devastated throughout New Orleans, especially the health- care safety net. This natural disaster revealed underlying vulnerabilities, as the New Orleans safety net was geographically and financially consolidated in the Medical Center of Louisiana at New Orleans (Charity Hospital). Charity Hospital was the central hub serving a patient population with complex health needs due to chronic disease, high rates of uninsured individuals, and high poverty rates. The damage from Hurricane Katrina meant that this safety net no longer functioned, and the city had to completely rebuild it. Rather than rebuild a single, centralized, and vulnerable hospital, the city invested in a network of primary-care clinics across the city that provide team-based care and integrate mental health with primary care, addressing the multiple factors affecting a person's health. This networked approach increases the resilience of the safety net, thereby improving its ability to withstand future disasters, and improves the preparedness of the community overall. Many of the important activities performed by the clinic network were supported by Federal grants and philanthropy, since current payment models do not reward these actions financially. The future of this initiative depends on an improved payment system, or the results will be unsustainable (see Goal 1).[46]

> **BOX 7. ASSISTING COMMUNITIES USING SYSTEMS APPROACHES—RETHINK HEALTH**[49]
>
> One example of using systems approaches at the community level is ReThink Health, which worked with local health leaders in Pueblo, Colorado to model all parts of the health-care system and all factors influencing health in a community. (Pueblo is a small county where 40 percent of residents are poor or unemployed, 1 in 6 is uninsured, and there are poor health outcomes for those with heart disease, diabetes, and other illnesses.) The community leaders used this model to consider the effectiveness of different policy strategies, identify potential bottlenecks or unsustainable funding, and understand the timeline for results. After using the model, community leaders put together a suite of policies to address the many underlying factors affecting problems facing their community, such as obesity and unintended pregnancy. This work is at an early stage, and the evaluation is ongoing. Knowledge has been gained in the process of community-wide decision making, such as the importance of involving groups beyond the traditional health-care system and the need for multiple policies to address the many factors affecting health.

## Opportunities Exist for Expanding Community Engagement in Health-Care Delivery

New delivery-system models and payment programs offer an opportunity to engage communities and states around systems-engineering approaches for improving health-care delivery. The State Innovation Model grants from CMS have provided a strong platform for improvement and reengineering health-care operations, and the Community-based Care Transitions Program brings together community stakeholders to reduce hospital readmissions for high-risk Medicare patients.[50] These are only examples of the multiple programs currently underway, with more being tested by the CMS Innovation Center that could be leveraged.

Another opportunity is to build upon the infrastructure created by the Beacon Community Program, which sought to demonstrate the potential for population-based health improvement by leveraging health IT and redesigning care delivery processes.[51] For example, the Southeast Minnesota Beacon Community wanted to develop new capabilities for exchanging data across its community. As part of its planning process, it convened a diverse group of stakeholders within the community (public-health departments, school districts, long-term care facilities, a statewide quality-performance-measures consumer organization,[52] and health-care organizations) and was able to adopt a comprehensive strategy. This strategy included expansion of EHR use among providers in public health departments, development of standard ways to capture and exchange continuity-of-care information, and establishment of a network for transferring health information between health-care providers. As a result, these new data capabilities provide tools for multiple organizations across the community to help keep people healthy.[53] The Southeast Minnesota Beacon Community, as well as its peers across the country, demonstrated that expanding health-IT infrastructure requires a strong governance system that incorporates stakeholder perspectives across the community to promote buy-in and coordinate across organizations.[54]

Community health needs assessments can generate incentives for partnerships with the community. These assessments help organizations understand the health needs of a community, such as a hospital's service area, a county, or region. Examples of current programs in this area include:

- The Affordable Care Act (ACA) requires tax-exempt hospitals to conduct a community health-needs assessment every three years and to update every year their implementation strategy to address targeted needs.
- The Centers for Disease Control and Prevention (CDC), in conjunction with the Robert Wood Johnson Foundation, supports the voluntary accreditation of local and State health departments through the Public Health Accreditation Board (PHAB). As part of gaining accreditation, the Board requires that departments conduct community health assessments.
- Community health centers are required to understand and address the health status and medical needs of vulnerable populations in their service areas as a condition for taking part in Federal programs or incentives for community health centers.

These assessments could be leveraged to increase the use of systems methods and tools. For example, requirements and guidelines could be revised so that the community is considered from a systems perspective, systems-engineering initiatives are conducted with partners in their communities, and sprogress is measured across the entire community in a systematic method. These requirements could be combined with technical assistance and resources to help with capacity-building in systems-engineering processes (see section on technical assistance). Combined with other recommendations, this expansion of needs-assessment activities could catalyze a powerful grassroots set of systems-engineering activities nationally, including hospitals, provider organizations, health departments, local foundations and non-profits, employers, schools, and many other stakeholders at local and regional levels.

**Recommendation 5**: Support efforts to engage the community in systematic health-care improvement.

- 5.1. Health and Human Services (HHS) should continue to support State and local efforts to transform health-care systems to provide better care quality and overall value.
- 5.2. Future Center for Medicare and Medicaid Services (CMS) Innovation Center programs should, as appropriate, incorporate systems-engineering principles at the community level; set, assess, and achieve population-level goals; and encourage grantees to engage stakeholders outside of the traditional health-care system.
- 5.3. HHS should leverage existing community needs assessment and planning processes, such as the community health-needs assessments for non-profit hospitals, ACO standards, health-department accreditation, and community health- center needs assessments, to promote systems thinking at the community level.

# GOAL 5. SHARE LESSONS LEARNED FROM SUCCESSFUL IMPROVEMENT EFFORTS

Some organizations are successfully using systems engineering to improve their operations, but the knowledge they have gained is not widely shared. These organizations have developed new improvement tools, identified the resources and circumstances needed for implementation, and uncovered the barriers that may limit success. Communicating the lessons learned can accelerate the efforts of those just beginning their system improvement efforts.

More research is needed to develop evidence about what works. Several Federal agencies have supported research on systems-engineering approaches—for example, the Agency for Health Research and Quality (AHRQ) has supported research on industrial and systems engineering in health care, and the National Science Foundation (NSF) and AHRQ have supported research on systems modeling to improve health systems. Beyond Federal programs, the Patient-Centered Outcomes Research Institute (PCORI) has announced initiatives aimed at improving health-care systems through engineering principles, and private foundations are also investing in these efforts. Further research could help uncover new knowledge, while expanded communication efforts could ensure the results are applied broadly.

There is another opportunity to learn what works through Federal programs that directly provide clinical care, such as the Veterans Health Administration (VHA) and Defense Health Agency (DHA). The VHA was an early leader in applications of systems engineering, and DHA has similarly leveraged systems methods and tools for serious conditions, such as traumatic brain injury. Greater dissemination of the knowledge gained from these practical experiences could assist more organizations in systems methods and tools.

One important dissemination channel is through convening and learning collaboratives. The Hospital Engagement Networks for the Partnership for Patients provides this type of learning collaborative for sharing best practices,[55] while the Center for Medicare and Medicaid Services (CMS) Innovation Centers offer a learning and diffusion group using a wide range of techniques to enable learning on a broad scale. Another example of collaborative approaches is the multi-state collaborative supported by the Milbank Memorial Fund. The goal of the collaborative is to support practices as they transition to Patient-Centered Medical Homes (PCMHs), a model of primary care that seeks to be patient-centered, comprehensive, coordinated, and accessible. The project brings together State- convened multi-payer PCMH efforts to share best practices and promote collaborative learning, encourage alignment in the PCMH programs offered by different payers, and support common evaluation and quality improvement.

Another useful way to share lessons learned is by using awards and prizes. Awards can provide an incentive by improving an organization's reputation, by a financial incentive attached to the award, or both. Beyond the incentive to participate, prizes and awards also provide an inventory of what works. There are already examples in health care where prizes promote action in important areas, such as the Monroe E. Trout Premier Cares Award to recognize organizations that support people excluded by or underserved by the traditional health-care system or the American Hospital Association NOVA Awards that acknowledge programs improving the health of the community.[56] There are opportunities to use awards and prizes to expand systems engineering in health care, building on existing ones—like the Shingo Prize[57] and Baldrige award (see Box 8)—that raise awareness of performance excellence.

> ## BOX 8. RECOGNIZING SUCCESSFUL USE OF SYSTEMS ENGINEERING— BALDRIGE PERFORMANCE EXCELLENCE PROGRAM[58]
>
> The National Institute of Standards and Technology (NIST) Baldrige Performance Excellence Program is a U.S. public-private partnership program designed to recognize and promote performance excellence. The program was established to identify and recognize high-performing companies, develop criteria for evaluating improvement efforts, and share best practices broadly. The Baldrige program raises awareness about the importance of performance improvement and provides tools and criteria to help organizations undertake that work. The program was expanded to include health-care and education organizations in 1999 and to nonprofit/government organizations in 2005.
>
> There are seven categories of criteria to help organizations identify their strengths and opportunities for improvement: leadership; strategic planning; customer focus; measurement, analysis, and knowledge management; workforce focus; operations focus; and results. The criteria focus on results—not procedures, tools, or organizational structure—in order to encourage creative, adaptive, and flexible approaches. Most importantly, the criteria support a systems perspective both to align goals across an organization and to encourage cycles of improvement with better feedback between improvement initiatives and its results.
>
> Over the past decade, an increasing proportion of these awards has been to health-care organizations. Last year, all of the winners were from the health-care and education sectors, which shows the appetite for improving the ways health care is organized and delivered.

**Recommendation 6**: Establish awards, challenges, and prizes to promote the use of systems methods and tools in health care.

6.1. Health and Human Services and the Department of Commerce should build on the Baldrige awards to recognize health-care providers successfully applying system engineering approaches.

## GOAL 6. TRAIN HEALTH PROFESSIONALS IN NEW SKILLS AND APPROACHES

Given changes in the way health care is delivered and an improved understanding of the many factors affecting a patient's health, health professionals of the future will need new skills to succeed. They will need effective communication and collaboration skills to work in teams, a commitment to lifelong learning to manage the flow of new evidence, and an appreciation and understanding of routine improvement methods. Expertise in systems engineering is especially critical as such tools can rarely be applied in a cookbook fashion, but rather need to be tailored to local circumstances to have the greatest chance of success.

Because systems science and systems engineering are central to improving health outcomes and health care's performance, system sciences and systems engineering need to be much more firmly and formally embedded in the training of all health-care professionals. It is crucial that both the knowledge of systems science and the skills of implementing the principles in health care are emphasized.[59] To this end, education must involve opportunities for interprofessional problem-solving and for building capacity for collaboration that facilitates practice change.

At present, clinical education and training falls short of this vision. Most clinicians were not trained in using systems-engineering approaches, and many clinicians may not even recognize that systems methods and tools could be helpful for improving care. Yet there are reasons for optimism. Several universities are leading the way by incorporating systems engineering directly into the curriculum for health professionals of all kinds (see Box 9 for an example of integrating systems engineering in nursing education). In addition to training clinicians about systems engineering tools, there is an opportunity to teach engineers about applying their tools in a health care environment. Some institutions have started internship opportunities for undergraduate and graduate students to work in hospitals and health systems, and others have begun joint classes where engineers and clinicians learn together about applying engineering concepts to care.[60] More broadly, organizations such as the Accreditation Council on Graduate Medical Education (ACGME) have already taken steps under their New Accreditation System and the Clinical Learning Environment Review to spotlight the need for trainees to develop competence in systems-based patient safety and quality improvement related tools. The Association of American Medical Colleges (AAMC) is addressing the need to develop skills related to systems engineering in medical schools; the American Association of Colleges of Nursing (AACN) includes organizational and systems leadership as an essential element of nursing education, particularly at the graduate levels; the American Medical Association (AMA) has launched an Accelerating Change in Medical Education Initiative to expand training in systems based practice and practice based improvement; and multiple clinical certifying boards have included practice-improvement modules in their maintenance-of-certification process. These are all positive developments and lay the groundwork for further improvement.

---

**BOX 9. TRAINING NURSES IN SYSTEMS ENGINEERING**

Nurses practice in a variety of roles, and systems engineering informs all of those roles—from providing direct care, to overseeing quality improvement, to leading organizations. Nurses are well-positioned to lead and participate in systems improvement because of the coordinating role they play among the patient, family, and care team, which helps to ensure continuity. From a process-design perspective, nurses contribute to continuity and communication among the team, coordinate care across settings, provide patient and family education and coaching, and collect and evaluate quality data to improve outcomes.

Nursing schools have evolved to teach these important skills. For example, the Gordon and Betty Moore Foundation established the Betty Irene Moore School of Nursing at UC Davis in 2009, with the explicit mission to improve health systems and advance health through nursing leadership.[61] Here, nurses study for graduate degrees (MS and PhD) in Nursing Science and Health Care Leadership, in a core curriculum that emphasizes systems engineering, implementation science, leadership, organizational change theory, quality improvement, interprofessional collaboration, and stakeholder engagement.

> Master's degree students complete 1 year of fieldwork in health-care organizations designing and implementing systems improvement projects, applying didactic learning to real-world complex problems. Through this experience, they build skills in problem analysis, stakeholder engagement in defining the problem and designing the solution, and business and sustainability issues to ensure best practices endure. The PhD students frame research questions using principles of systems engineering and implementation science and tackle complex problems in health care and health. Early graduates of this program are assuming leadership positions, and several have successfully designed and now occupy new roles in health-care systems emphasizing quality improvement.

There are several policy options that build on existing Federal roles in education and training for physicians, nurses, pharmacists, physical therapists, behavioral health practitioners, health professionals, and health-care administrators. Current Federal education programs are diverse, ranging from loan repayment programs for practicing in medically underserved areas, supporting graduate medical education, and sponsoring continuing education events. The existing education programs could be leveraged to ensure more clinicians and others working in the health-care system have the needed skills and competencies in systems approaches.

**Recommendation 7**: Build competencies and workforce for redesigning health care.

- 7.1. Health and Human Services should use a wide range of funding, program, and partnership levers to educate clinicians about systems-engineering competencies for scalable health-care improvement.
- 7.2. HHS should collect, inventory, and disseminate best practices in curricular and learning activities, as well as encourage knowledge sharing through regional learning communities. These functions could be accomplished through the new extension-center functions.
- 7.3. HHS should create grant programs for developing innovative health-professional curricula that include systems engineering and implementation science, and HHS should disseminate the grant products broadly.
- 7.4. HHS should fund systems-engineering centers of excellence to build a robust specialty in Health Improvement Science for physicians, nurses, health professionals, and administrators.

## SUMMARY AND CONCLUSION

Given recent successes in expanding access to the health-care system, it is now time to ensure that all patients have access to safe, high quality, affordable care. One important tool for addressing these challenges is through systems engineering, which has improved quality, reliability, and overall value in other industries. These methods and tools have similar potential for health care, as evidenced by a small number of health-care organizations that have applied these principles to their own operations. There are several challenges that are limiting the spread of this concept—including technical and infrastructure, policy, cultural, and organizational barrier. Given the diverse challenges, this report identifies a comprehensive set of recommendations to encourage the use of systems engineering by:

1. Accelerating alignment of payment systems with desired outcomes,
2. Increasing access to relevant health data and analytics,
3. Providing technical assistance in systems-engineering approaches,
4. Involving communities in improving health-care delivery, and
5. Sharing lessons learned from successful improvement efforts,
6. Training health professionals in new skills and approaches.

By implementing these recommendations, which support and reinforce each other, systems approaches can become widely used tools for improving the health of all Americans while ensuring that health care remains affordable for families, businesses, and the Nation.

## APPENDIX A. SYSTEMS ENGINEERING OVERVIEW

*What is it?* An interdisciplinary approach to analyze, design, manage, and/or measure a complex system with efforts to improve it (through increased efficiency, productivity, quality, safety, and other factors).

*How are systems formed?* In the context of systems engineering, systems are interconnected elements (processes, people, products) that, when connected, form an entity (an organization, a finished good, a completed service).

- *Systems need boundaries.* System boundaries can be designed to include the entire system's life cycle (cradle to grave) or just single components (vehicle assembly line, patient-clinician in-office interaction).
- *Systems should be stakeholder-focused.* Systems should be developed by concentrating on (internal and/or external) stakeholder needs. System improvements should enhance (add value) to the impacted stakeholders.
- *Systems are data-driven.* Systems have clear measurable goals defined to assist with the analysis of the problem as well as impact of implemented solution. The outcomes of these goals are measured with data collected.

***How is it operationalized?*** System engineering processes typically include several sequential steps, leading from problem investigation to solution evaluation. Depending on the strategy taken to analyze the system, steps to operationalize can include:

- Problem/Needs Definition
- Modeling the System
- Analysis of Alternatives
- Implementation of Selected Alternative
- Assessment of Performance of Improved System

***What strategies are used for improvement?*** Different and multiple strategies can be used depending on the system characteristics (type, size, boundaries, etc.).

# APPENDIX B. SELECTED EXAMPLES OF SYSTEMS ENGINEERING IN HEALTH CARE

There are many examples where systems engineering has been applied to improve health care. This appendix describes some of these examples to illustrate the potential range and impact from these methods and tools.

## Redesigning a Hospital Pharmacy with Systems Engineering

Impacts can be similarly significant at a smaller scale. Figure B-1 illustrates the change in workflow that occurred after a systems-engineering intervention in one clinical pharmacy. Before, different people would go to the same place to search for filled prescriptions and materials, unbeknownst to each other, which led to waste in terms of motion and overprocessing. The systems-engineering effort identified several specific challenges, for which targeted changes were made, leading to a streamlined process, less overproduction waste, and reduced unnecessary motion.

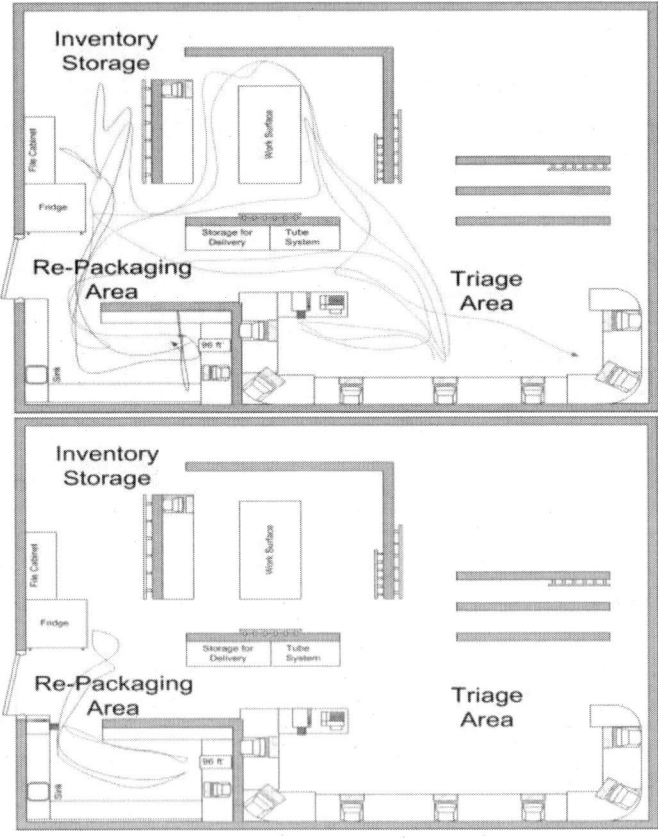

Figure B-1. Workflow in one pharmacy unit before (left) and after (right) systems-engineering methods were used.[62]

## Addressing Alcohol Abuse in San Francisco

The City and County of San Francisco saw very high rates of individuals coming to the emergency room with alcohol abuse events. To deal with this problem, the localities sought to re-engineer how the community handled alcohol abuse events, with the goal of reducing the frequency that alcohol-dependent people were treated by hospital emergency departments. To do so, they created "The Sobering Center," which serves as a physical place where inebriated individuals can rest while they are under the influence of alcohol. These individuals are referred to the Sobering Center by emergency services, police, social workers, and emergency departments, which requires collaboration among many different organizations to reconsider their processes. In terms of results, the Sobering Center has provided services to over 8,000 people, has prevented over 29,000 unnecessary emergency department visits and ambulance transports, and thereby has saved costs. Furthermore, it provides additional supports for the people using the Center by connecting them to other social-support services.[63]

## Coordinating Care across the Community: Vermont Blueprint for Health

The Vermont Blueprint for Health was created to improve health care delivery across the State and thereby improve people's health. This Statewide public-private initiative is organized around advanced primary care practices, which are recognized as patient centered medical homes by the National Committee for Quality Assurance (NCQA). Recognizing that most practices in the State are small, the Blueprint supports each practice with robust health information technology and multi-disciplinary community health teams. These locally-based teams bring together professionals from social work, nursing, and behavioral health help to coordinate care for all patients, identify those with the greatest health needs, and ensure that all are able to manage their health. This project is supported by all payers in Vermont—including Medicaid, Medicare, and private payers—to ensure funding remains sustainable. The Blueprint has seen favorable outcomes for patients helped by both the medical homes and community health teams. In 2012, those patients had lower health care expenditures (20 percent less for children, 10 percent less for adults younger than age 65), were more likely to receive evidence-based preventive services, and were less likely to be hospitalized. The Blueprint continues its work and is expanding further in the State.[64]

# APPENDIX C. GLOSSARY

**Agile Management:** flexible approach focused on understanding stakeholder needs through incremental, iterative changes in the system; changes are evaluated after each implementation to determine next steps. Common tools include wikis and project-management software.

**Business Process Management:** cross-functional, iterative approach to optimize processes and knowledge transfers as changes occur in the system. Most common tools are software packages (vendors include IBM, Oracle) implemented to manage workflows, documents, and processes.

**Complexity Science**: study of how "Complex Adaptive Systems" perform and what influences their behavior. Because some parts of the system are "animate" – or respond on their own to inputs and the environment – human systems tend to be "complex" and "adaptive," which has implications for how they are managed.

**Human Factors**: study of the cognitive and environmental influences on human performance.

**Lean Enterprise System:** holistic approach focused on removal of "wastes" in the entire product life cycle; emphasizes continuous improvement, organizational learning, and dynamic process flows. Common tools include kaizen "improve for better" events and value-stream mapping. Also known as Toyota Production System, just-in- time (JIT) manufacturing.

**Lean Six Sigma**: combination of Lean Enterprise System and Six Sigma best practices; emphasizes using problem- solving Six Sigma tools to remove wastes identified in Lean.

**Microsystem**: system nested within a larger system. In health care, this could include a critical care unit, emergency response network, or blood bank inside a larger health care organization. A challenge is that a microsystem may be optimally functioning for its own purposes, but the larger organization may have poorer performance because it does not consider how the individual microsystems work together.

**Performance Improvement**: measurable improvement (intent) of functioning systems (context) of care. It is frequently not possible to "control" the environment of or multiple inputs into these functional systems or understand the impact of all the combinations and permutations of the inputs.

**Process Improvement**: sciences of improving system performance including methods such as Lean and Six-Sigma.

**Quality Management:** see performance improvement.

**Queuing Theory, Flow, and the Theory of Constraints**: study of how people and materials move or flow through a system.

**Reliability And Maintainability**: study of high reliability in system design and performance and its determinants and requirements.

**Six Sigma**: formalized approach to reduce variation with defined operational steps to problem-solving (using the DMAIC model – Define, Measure, Analyze, Improve, Control). Popularized by Motorola and GE. Common tools include cause and effect "fishbone" diagrams, sigma calculations, and control charts.

**Statistical Process Control**: science of measuring system performance over time.

**System**: set of interdependent parts that share a common purpose. There are 3 key aspects of this definition. First, a system shares a common purpose or goals. Second, the system is made up of several parts. Third, the parts are interdependent. There are systems, often termed systems of systems, where the component systems have conflicting goals. Health care delivery is such a system.

**Systems engineering**: interdisciplinary field that designs and manages complex projects (systems) over their life cycles. It consider issues such as system purpose, architecture, environment, materials reliability, logistics, work- processes, optimization methods, risk management, coordination of different teams, evaluation measurements, cost, schedule, and much more, all of which gains complexity when dealing with large, complex projects or systems.

**Systems science**: study of system performance with the objective of system performance improvement. In health care, this would mean achieving better results for patients. System science is an interdisciplinary field incorporating systems engineering; social sciences; complexity science; queuing theory, flow, and the theory of constraints; human factors; reliability and maintainability; process improvement; and statistical process control.

## APPENDIX D. ABBREVIATIONS

| | |
|---|---|
| **AAMC** | Association of American Medical Colleges |
| **ACA** | Patient Protection and Affordable Care Act |
| **ACGME** | Accreditation Council for Graduate Medical Education |
| **ACO** | Accountable Care Organization |
| **AHA** | American Hospital Association |
| **AHRQ** | Agency for Healthcare Research and Quality |
| **AMA** | American Medical Association |
| **ARRA** | American Recovery and Reinvestment Act |
| **CDC** | Centers for Disease Control & Prevention |
| **CMS** | Centers for Medicare & Medicaid Services |
| **DoD** | Department of Defense |
| **DOE** | Department of Energy |
| **EHR** | Electronic Health Record |
| **EIA** | Energy Information Administration |
| **FDA** | Food and Drug Administration |
| **GAO** | Government Accountability Office |
| **HIE** | Health Information Exchange |
| **HITECH** | Health Information Technology for Economic and Clinical Health Act |
| **HHS** | U.S. Department of Health and Human Services |
| **HRSA** | Health Resources and Services Administration |
| **IOM** | Institute of Medicine |
| **JASON** | An independent scientific advisory group that provides consulting services to the U.S. government on matters of defense science and technology. It was established in 1960. The name of the group is not an acronym. |
| **MEP** | Hollings Manufacturing Extension Partnership |
| **NIH** | National Institutes of Health |
| **NIST** | National Institute of Standards and Technology |
| **NSF** | National Science Foundation |
| **ONC** | Office of the National Coordinator for Health Information Technology |
| **PCORI** | Patient Centered Outcomes Research Institute |
| **PCMH** | Patient Centered Medical Home |
| **PHAB** | Public Health Accreditation Board |
| **QIO** | Quality Improvement Organization |

| | |
|---|---|
| **REC** | Regional Extension Center |
| **TQM** | Total Quality Management |
| **VHA** | Veterans Health Administration |

# APPENDIX E. 2010 PCAST REPORT ON HEALTH INFORMATION TECHNOLOGY

*This report describes several recommendations to support an operational national health IT infrastructure. Those recommendations for Federal agencies are listed below.*[65]

The Chief Technology Officer of the United States should:

- In coordination with the Office of Management and Budget (OMB) and the Secretary of HHS, and using technical expertise within ONC, develop within 12 months a set of metrics that measure progress toward an operational, universal, national health IT infrastructure. Research, prototype, and pilot efforts should not be included in this metric of operational progress.
- Annually, assess the Nation's progress in health IT by the metrics developed, and make recommendations to OMB and the Secretary of HHS on how to make more rapid progress.

The Office of the National Coordinator should:

- Move more boldly to ensure that the Nation has electronic health systems that are able to exchange health data in a universal manner based on metadata-tagged data elements. In particular, ONC should signal now that systems will need to have this capability by 2013 in order to be deemed as making "meaningful use" of electronic health information under the HITECH Act.
- Act to establish initial minimal standards for the metadata associated with tagged data elements, and develop a roadmap for more complete standards over time.
- Facilitate the rapid mapping of existing semantic taxonomies into tagged data elements, while continuing to encourage the longer-term harmonization of these taxonomies by vendors and other stakeholders.

- Support the development of reference implementations for the use of tagged data elements in products. Certification of individual products should focus on interoperability with the reference implementations.
- Set standards for the necessary data element access services (specifically, indexing and access control) and formulate a strategic plan for bringing such services into operation in an interoperable and intercommunicating manner. Immediate priority should be given to those services needed to locate data relating to an individual patient.
- Facilitate, with the Small Business Administration, the emergence of competitive companies that would provide small or under-resourced physician practices, community-based long-term care facilities, and hospitals with a range of cloud-based services.
- Ensure that research funded through the SHARP (Strategic Health IT Advanced Research Projects) program on data security include the use of metadata to enable data security.

The Centers for Medicare & Medicaid Services should:

- Redirect the focus of meaningful use measures as rapidly as possible from data collection of specified lists of health measures to higher levels of data exchange and the increased use of clinical decision supports.
- Direct its efforts under the Patient Protection and Affordable Care Act toward the ability to receive and use data from multiple sources and formats.
- In parallel with (i.e., without waiting for) the NRC study on IT modernization, begin to develop options for the modernization and full integration of its information systems platforms using modern technologies, and with the necessary transparency to build confidence with Congress and other stakeholders.
- When informed by the preliminary and final NRC study reports, move rapidly to implement one or more of the options already formulated, or formulate new options as appropriate, with the goal of making substantial progress by 2013 and completing implementation by 2014. CMS must transition into a modern information technology organization, allowing integration of multiple components and consistent use of standards and processes across all the provider sectors and programs it manages.

- Exercise its influence as the Nation's largest healthcare payer to accelerate the implementation of health information exchange using tagged data elements. By 2013, meaningful use criteria should include data submitted through reference implementation processes, either directly to CMS or (if CMS modernization is not sufficiently advanced) through private entities authorized to serve this purpose.
- By 2013, provide incentives for hospitals and eligible professionals to submit meaningful use clinical measures that are calculated from computable data. By 2015, encourage or require that quality measures under all of its reporting programs (the Physician Quality Reporting Initiative, hospitals, Medicare Advantage plans, nursing homes, etc.) be able to be collected in a tagged data element model.

The Department of Health and Human Services should:

- Develop a strategic plan for rapid action that integrates and aligns information systems through the government's public health agencies (including FDA, CDC, NIH, and AHRQ) and benefits payment systems (CMS and VA).
- Convene a high-level task force to align data standards, and population research data, between private and public sector payers.
- Convene a high-level task force to develop specific recommendations on national standards that enable patient access, data exchange, and de-identified data aggregation for research purposes, in a model based on tagged data elements that embed privacy rules, policies and applicable patient preferences in the metadata traveling with each data element.
- As the necessary counterpart to technical security measures, propose an appropriate structure of administrative, civil, and criminal penalties for the misuse of a national health IT infrastructure and individual patient records, wherever such data may reside.
- Appoint a working group of diverse expert stakeholders to develop policies and standards for the appropriate secondary uses of healthcare data. This could be tasked to the Interagency Coordinating Council for Comparative Effectiveness Research.
  - With FDA, bring about the creation of a trusted third-party notification service that would identify and implement methods for reidentification of individuals when data analysis produces important new findings.

Other or multiple agencies:

- AHRQ should be funded to develop a test network for comparative effectiveness research. The FDA, and also other HHS public health agencies, should enable medical researchers to gain access to de-identified, aggregated, near-real-time medical data by using data element access services.
- HHS should coordinate ONC activities with CDC, FDA, and any other entities developing adverse event and syndromic surveillance networks.
- The Department of Defense and the Department of Veteran Affairs should engage with ONC and help to drive the development of standards for universal data exchange of which they can become early adopters.

# APPENDIX F. 2014 JASON REPORT ON HEALTH DATA INFRASTRUCTURE

*This report discusses benefits of and challenges to enhancing health-data infrastructure. Findings and recommendations are presented below.*[66]

## Findings

1. The current lack of interoperability among data resources for EHRs is a major impediment to the unencumbered exchange of health information and the development of a robust health data infrastructure. Interoperability issues can be resolved only by establishing a comprehensive, transparent, and overarching software architecture for health information.
2. The twin goals of improved health care and lowered health care costs will be realized only if health- related data can be explored and exploited in the public interest, for both clinical practice and

   biomedical research. That will require implementing technical solutions that both protect patient privacy and enable data integration across patients.

3. The criteria for Stage 1 and Stage 2 Meaningful Use, while surpassing the 2013 goals set forth by HHS for EHR adoption, fall short of achieving meaningful use in any practical sense. At present, large-scale interoperability amounts to little more than replacing fax machines with the electronic delivery of page- formatted medical records. Most patients still cannot gain electronic access to their health information. Rational access to EHRs for clinical care and biomedical research does not exist outside the boundaries of individual organizations.
4. Although current efforts to define standards for EHRs and to certify HIT systems are useful, they lack a unifying software architecture to support broad interoperability. Interoperability is best achieved through the development of a comprehensive, open architecture.
5. Current approaches for structuring EHRs and achieving interoperability have largely failed to open up new opportunities for entrepreneurship and innovation that can lead to products and services that enhance health care provider workflow and strengthen the connection between the patient and the health care system, thus impeding progress toward improved health outcomes.
6. HHS has the opportunity to drive adoption and interoperability of electronic health records by defining successive stages of Meaningful Use criteria that move progressively from the current closed box systems to an open software architecture.
7. The biomedical research community will be a major consumer of data from an interoperable health data infrastructure. At present, access to health data is mostly limited to proprietary datasets of selected patients. Broad access to health data for research purposes is essential to realizing the long-term benefits of a robust health data infrastructure.
8. The data contained in EHRs will increase tremendously, both in volume and in the diversity of input sources. It will include genomic and other "omic" data, self-reported data from embedded and wireless sensors, and data gleaned from open sources. Some types of personal health data, especially when combined, will make it possible to decipher the identity of the individual, even when the data are stripped of explicit identifying information, thus raising challenges for maintaining patient privacy.

9. The US population is highly diverse, reflecting much of the diversity of the global population. Therefore, important research findings applicable to Americans are likely to come from shared access to international health data. Currently there is no coherent mechanism for accessing such data for research.
10. Electronic access to health data will make it easier to identify fraudulent activity, but at present there is little effort to do so using EHRs.

## Recommendations

1. CMS should embrace Stage 3 Meaningful Use as an opportunity to break free from the status quo and embark upon the creation of a truly interoperable health data infrastructure.
2. An immediate goal, to be sought within 12 months (including time for consultation with stakeholders), should be for ONC to define an overarching software architecture for the health data infrastructure.
   2.1. The architecture should provide a logical organization of functions that allow interoperability, protect patient privacy, and facilitate access for clinical care and biomedical research. JASON has provided an example of what such an architecture might look like.
   2.2. The architecture should identify the small set of necessary interfaces between functions, recognizing that the purpose of a software architecture is to provide structure, while avoiding having "everything talking to everything."
   2.3. The architecture should be defined, but not necessarily implemented, within the 12 month period. During that time, ONC should create (or redirect) appropriate committees to carry out, continuing beyond the 12 month horizon, the detailed development of requirements for the functions and interfaces that comprise the architecture.
3. To achieve the goal of improving health outcomes, Stage 3 Meaningful Use requirements should be defined such that they enable the creation of an entrepreneurial space across the entire health data enterprise.

3.1. EHR software vendors should be required to develop and publish APIs for medical records data, search and indexing, semantic harmonization and vocabulary translation, and user interface applications. In addition, they should be required to demonstrate that data from their EHRs can be exchanged through the use of these APIs and used in a meaningful way by third-party software developers.
3.2. The APIs should be certified through vetting by multiple third-party developers in regularly scheduled "code-a-thons."
3.3. Commercial system acquisition by the VA and DOD should adhere to the requirements for creating public APIs, publishing and vetting them, and demonstrating meaningful data exchange by third- party software developers.
4. The ONC should solicit input from the biomedical research community to ensure that the health data infrastructure meets the needs of researchers. This would be best accomplished by convening a meeting of representative researchers within the immediate (12 month) time frame for architecture definition.
5. The adopted software architecture must have the flexibility to accommodate new data types that will be generated by emerging technologies, the capacity to expand greatly in size, and the ability to balance the privacy implications of new data types with the societal benefits of biomedical research.
6. The ONC should exert leadership in facilitating international interoperability for health data sharing for research purposes. The genomics community is already engaged in such efforts for the sharing of sequence data, and the ONC should consider adopting a similar process.
7. Large-scale data mining techniques and predictive analytics should be employed to uncover signatures of fraud. A data enclave should be established to support the ongoing development and validation of fraud detection tools to maintain their effectiveness as fraud strategies evolve.

# APPENDIX G. ILLUSTRATIVE EXAMPLES ON WAYS TO BUILD HHS DATA LEADERSHIP

Infrastructure and Governance

- Appoint chief data officers for key agencies, reporting to agency executive.
- Treat data on health system performance as a core national business asset including better data governance and strategic investments in data analysis, methods, tools, partnerships and staff.
- Have direct hiring authority to bring on key staff (data science, technology).

Data Innovation and Engagement

- Continue and accelerate HHS open data activities (dissemination, engagement with private sector, user- friendly tools).
- Develop user-friendly data products and tools targeted to groups driving health system improvement
- (providers, consumer groups, employers, state leaders, health plans, companies)
- Accelerate release of data on health system performance (quality, safety, cost) at the provider, regional and state level, including appropriate benchmarks.
- Expand access to Medicare claims and other high-value data sets beyond currently defined research and quality-reporting purposes and at an affordable cost.
- Invest in data methods, tools and standards that permit linking and analysis of identifiable data sets without exposing personal health information (PHI).
- Hire data scientists and engineers to create internal HHS resources and infrastructure.
- Demonstrate how HHS data are fueling new innovations, entrepreneurship and low-cost technologies to improve HHS' efficiency, effectiveness and performance.
- Invite data insights and discovery from across HHS and public (challenges, crowd-sourcing discovery).

- Develop data partnerships to support developing and sharing data sets with linked government and private sector data.

Data-Driven Performance

- Increase investments in analysis, management and dissemination of data relative to data collection in support of systems engineering.
- Link and compile data from across HHS and from outside sources to better track health care delivery system performance.
- Develop business intelligence tools which mine existing data to provide real-time tracking of health care delivery system performance, identify areas of improvement that should be tapped to figure out and disseminate what's working and pinpoint areas of lagging performance that need to be explored and addressed. These data should drive HHS business decisions, budgets and dissemination activities.

## APPENDIX H. ADDITIONAL EXPERTS PROVIDING INPUT

**Scott Anderson**
Director of Quality
GE Healthcare

**Anne-Marie J. Audet**
Vice President, Delivery System Reform and
Breakthrough Opportunities
The Commonwealth Fund

**Richard Baron**
President and CEO
American Board of Internal Medicine

**John Beasley**
Faculty
University of Wisconsin School of Medicine and
Public Health

**Maureen Bisognano**
CEO
Institute for Healthcare Improvement

**George Wong Bo-Linn**
Chief Program Officer, Patient Care Program
Gordon and Betty Moore Foundation

**Jason Boehm**
Director, Program Coordination Office
Chief of Staff
U.S. Department of Commerce

**Albert Bonnema**
Chief Medical Information Officer
Air Force Medical Services

**Franklin E. Bragg**
Physician
Bangor Beacon Community Medical Center and
Eastern Main Medical Center

**Jennifer L. Brull**
Physician and Owner
Prairie Star Family Practice

**Sean Cavanaugh**
Deputy Director of Programs and Policy, Center for
Medicare and Medicaid Innovation
Centers for Medicare and Medicaid Services (CMS)

**Patrick H. Conway**
Chief Medical Officer, Centers for Medicare and
Medicaid Services (CMS)
Director, Center for Clinical Standards and Quality

**Theresa A. Cullen**
Director, Health Informatics
U.S. Department of Veterans Affairs

**Samuel Cykert**
Clinical Director, North Carolina Regional Extension center and Interim Director, University of North Carolina School of Medicine Health Informatics Program

**Ivor Douglas**
Chief, Pulmonary Sciences & Critical Care
Medicine Director, Medical Intensive Care
Denver Health Medical Center

**James Doyle**
Vice President of 300mm Operations, Systems and Technology Group, Packaging, Assembly and Test IBM

**William Ike Eisenhaur**
National Director of Veterans Engineering Resource Centers
Veteran's Health Administration

**Yul D. Ejnes**
Private Practice Internist, Coastal Medical Inc.
Chair-Emeritus, Board of Regents, American College of Physicians

**Susan Dentzer**
Senior Policy Adviser
Robert Wood Johnson Foundation

**Robert Fangmeyer**
Acting Director
Baldrige Performance Excellence Program
National Institute of Standards and Technology

**Bruce Goldberg**
Director
Oregon Health Authority

**Donald Goldmann**
Chief Medical and Scientific Officer
Institute for Healthcare Improvement

**Patrick Gordon**
Associate Vice President, Community Integration
Rocky Mountain Health Plans

**Oren Grad**
Consultant
IDA Science and Technology Policy Institute

**Judith A. Hautala**
Research Staff Member
IDA Science and Technology Policy Institute

**Robin Hemphill**
Doctor of Emergency Medicine
Vanderbilt University Medical Center

**Carlos Roberto Jaen**
Professor and Chairman, Department of Family and Community Medicine
University of Texas Health Science Center at San Antonio

**Brent James**
Executive Director, Institute for Health Care
Delivery and Research
Vice President of Medical Research and Continuing Medical Education,
Intermountain Healthcare

**Robert L. Jesse**
Principal Deputy Under Secretary for Health Department of Veterans Affairs

**Craig A. Jones**
Director, Vermont Blueprint for Health
State of Vermont

**Michael Kanter**
Medical Director of Quality and Clinical Analysis Southern California Kaiser Permanente Medical Group

**Anita Karcz**
Chief Medical officer
Institute for Health Metrics

**Neva Kaye**
Managing Director for Health System Performance
National Academy for Sate Health Policy (NASHP)

**Sallie Ann Keller**
Director and Professor of Statistics, Virginia
Bioinformatics Institute
Virginia Tech University

**Janhavia Kirtain**
Director of Clinical Transformation
Beacon Community Cooperative Agreement Program

**Paul Kleeberg**
Chief Medical Informatics Officer, Stratis Health Clinical Director for REACH, the Regional Extension Assistance Center for HIT

**Shari M. Ling**
Deputy Chief Medical Officer, Center for Clinical Standards and Quality
Centers for Medicare and Medicaid Services (CMS)

**Mark McClellan**
Director and Senior Fellow, Health Care Innovation and Value Initiative
Engelberg Center for Health Care Reform, Brookings Institution

**Terry McGeeney**
Director
BDC Advisors

**Elizabeth McGlynn**
Director
Kaiser Permanente Center for Effectiveness & Safety Research (CESR)

**Bobby Milstein**
Director
ReThink Health

**Mark Monroe**
Senior Director of Risk Management
Kaiser Permanente

**Farzad Mostashari**
Visiting Fellow
Engelberg Center for Health Care Reform, Brookings Institution

**Richard Newall**
Gendell Professor of Energy and Environment
Economics and Director
Duke University Energy Initiative

**Sean Nolan**
Chief Architect and General Manager
Health Solutions Group, Microsoft Corporation

**Samuel R. Nussbaum**
Executive Vice President for Clinical Health Policy and Chief Medical Officer, WellPoint, Inc.

**Margaret E. O'Kane**
President
National Committee for Quality Assurance

**James C. Puffer**
President and Chief Executive Officer
American Board of Family Medicine

**Proctor Reid**
Director of Programs
National Academic of Engineering

**Lewis G. Sandy**
Executive Vice President for Clinical Advancement
UnitedHealth Group

**Judy Schilz**
Director of Care Delivery Transformation
WellPoint, Inc.

**Bryan T. Scott**
Director of Quality, St. Louis Site
Boeing Defense Space and Security

**Martin Sepulveda**
Vice President of Integrated Health Services
IBM Corporation

**Phillip Singerman**
Acting Director
Hollings Manufacturing Extension Partnership
National Institute of Standards and Technology

**Christine A. Sinsky**
Internal Medicine Physician
Medical Associates Clinic and Health Plans

**Ida Sim**
Professor
University of California at San Francisco School of Medicine

**William W. Stead**
McKesson Foundation Professor of Biomedical Informatics
Vanderbilt University

**Jonathan R. Sugarman**
President and CEO Qualis Health

**Margaret Van Amringe**
Executive Vice President of Public Policy and Government Relations
The Joint Commission

**Henry Wei**
Presidential Innovation Fellow
Senior Medical Director, Clinical Innovation Aetna

**Jonathan Woodson**
Assistant Secretary of Defense (Health Affairs) and Director
Tricare Management Activity

**Scott Young**
Associate Executive Director for Clinical Care and Innovation, The Permanente Federation, LLC Senior Medical Director and Executive Director, Care Management Institute

**Teresa Zayas Caban**
Chief of Health IT Research
Agency for Healthcare Research

# End Notes

[1] Patient Protection and Affordable Care Act, 42 U.S.C. § 18001 (2010).

[2] See, for *Best Care at Lower cost: The Path to Continuously Learning Health Care in America*, Washington, DC: National Academies Press, 2012.

[3] Institute of Medicine. *Crossing the Quality Chasm: A New Health System for the 21st Century*, Washington, DC: The National Academies Press, 2001.

[4] (1) Levinson, D. R. "Adverse events in hospitals: National incidence among Medicare beneficiaries," Washington, D.C.: U.S. Department of Health and Human Services, Office of Inspector General, 2010. (2) Levinson, D.R. "Hospital incident reporting systems do not capture most patient harm," Washington, D.C.: U.S. Department of Health and Human Services, Office of Inspector General, 2012. (3) Classen, D. C., et al. "'Global trigger tool' shows that adverse events in hospitals may be ten times greater than previously measured," *Health Affairs* (Millwood) 30(4):581-589, 2011. (4) Landrigan, C. P., et al. "Temporal trends in rates of patient harm resulting from medical care," *New England Journal of Medicine* 363(22):2124-2134, 2010.

[5] Wallace, C. J., and L. Savitz. "Estimating waste in frontline health care worker activities," *Journal of Evaluation in Clinical Practice* 14(1):178-180, 2008.

[6] American Recovery and Reinvestment Act (ARRA) of 2009, Pub. L. No. 111-5, 123 Stat. 115 (2009).

[7] The National Quality Strategy is described online at: http://www.ahrq.gov/workingforquality/

[8] Lewis, G. H., et al. "Counterheroism, Common Knowledge, and Ergonomics: Concepts from Aviation That Could Improve Patient Safety," *Milbank Quarterly*, 89:4–38, 2011.

[9] See, for example: Rouse, W.B. and W.D. Compton. "Systems Engineering and Management," *Engineering the Systems of Healthcare Delivery*, ed. W.B. Rouse and D.A. Cortese, Amsterdam: IOS Press, 2010.

[10] (1) Kaplan, Gary, et al. *Bringing a Systems Approach to Health*, National Academy of Engineering and Institute of Medicine Systems Approaches to Improving Health Innovation

Collaborative, Washington, DC. http://www.iom.edu/~/media/Files/Perspectives-Files/2013/Discussion-Papers/VSRT-SAHIC-Overview.pdf. (2) Schultz, Rebecca and Elena Simoncini. "Combating Hospital Noise and False Alarms Through Clinical Engineering and Nursing Collaboration." http://www.accenet.org/downloads/reference/StudentPaper-Winner%202012.pdf

[11] According to the Clinical Outcomes Report produced by University Health System Consortium, the observed mortality rate at Denver Health decreased to 1.17%. See: http://www.denverhealth.org/medical-services/trauma-center/choose-denver- health

[12] See for example: (1) Meyer, H. "Life in the 'Lean' lane: Performance improvement at Denver Health," *Health Affairs* 29(11):2054-2060, 2010. (2) Gabow, P.A. and P.S. Mehler. "A broad and structured approach to improving patient safety and quality: lessons from Denver Health," *Health Affairs* 30(4):612-618, 2011. (3) Gabow, P. "The promise of lean processes," *IOM Commentary,* Washington, DC: Institute of Medicine, 2012.

[13] (1) Schilling, L., et al. "Kaiser Permanente's Performance Improvement System, Part 1: From Benchmarking to Executing on Strategic Priorities," *The Joint Commission Journal on Quality and Patient Safety* 36(11): 484-498, 2010. (2) Schilling, L., et al. "Kaiser Permanente's Performance Improvement System, Part 2: Developing a Value Framework," *The Joint Commission Journal on Quality and Patient Safety* 36(12):552-560, 2010.

[14] (1) Crawford, B., et al. "Kaiser Permanente Northern California sepsis mortality reduction initiative," *Critical Care*, 16(Suppl 3):P12, 2012. (2) Whippy, A., et al. "Kaiser Permanente's Performance Improvement System, Part 3: Multisite Improvements in Care for Patients with Sepsis," *Joint Commission Journal on Quality and Patient Safety*, 37(11):483-493, 2011.

[15] Drawn from personal communication with Robert Dittus, Vanderbilt.

[16] (1) Roumie, Christianne L., et al. "Improving Blood Pressure Control through Provider Education, Provider Alerts, and Patient Education – A Cluster Randomized Trial," *Annals of Internal Medicine* 145(3): 165-175, 2006. (2) Choma, Neesha N., et al. "Quality improvement initiatives improve hypertension care among veterans." *Circulation: Cardiovascular Quality and Outcomes* 2(4): 392-398, 2009.

[17] According to a UnitedHealth Group working paper, "No national health policy prescription is complete without the exhortation to move from a health care system that pays for volume to one that pays for value." http://www.unitedhealthgroup.com/~/media/UHG/PDF/2012/UNH-Working-Paper-8.ashx

[18] (1) Bagian, J.P. "Patient safety: What is really at issue? *Frontiers of Health Services Management*." 22(1):3-16, 2005. (2) Neily, J., et al. "Association Between Implementation of a Medical Team Training Program and Surgical Mortality," *Journal of the American Medical Association*, 304(15):1693-1700, 2010.

[19] (1) Pronovost, P., et al. "An intervention to decrease catheter-related bloodstream infections in the ICU." *New England Journal of Medicine*, 355(26):2725-2732, 2006. (3) Pronovost, P., et al. "Creating high reliability in health care organizations," *Health Services Research* 41(4 Pt 2):1599-1617, 2006.

[20] 2012 American Medical Association (AMA) Physician Practice Benchmark Survey (PPBS).

[21] American Medical Association. "AMA Releases New Study of Physician Practice Arrangements," *AMA*, September 17, 2013, http://www.ama-assn.org/ama/pub/news/news/2013/2013-09-17-new-study-physician-practice- arrangements.page.

[22] 2012 American Medical Association (AMA) Physician Practice Benchmark Survey (PPBS).

[23] See for instance, McCannon, C.J. and A. McKethan. "How it's done: Keys to implementation of delivery system reform," *Healthcare*, 1(3-4):69-71, 2013.

[24] Hsu, E., et al. "Doing Well by Doing Good: Assessing the Cost Savings of an Intervention to Reduce Central Line–Associated Bloodstream Infections in a Hawaii Hospital," *American Journal of Medical Quality*, 29(1):13-19, 2014.

[25] (1) Pham, H. H., et al. "Redesigning care delivery in response to a high-performance network: The Virginia Mason Medical Center," *Health Affairs*, 26(4):w532-w544, 2007. (2)

Ginsburg, P.B., et al. "Distorted payment system undermines business case for health quality and efficiency gains," Issue Brief, Center for the Study of Health System Change (112):1-4, 2007. (3) Blackmore, C. C., et al. "At Virginia Mason, collaboration among providers, employers, and health plans to transform care cut costs and improved quality," *Health Affairs* 30(9):1680-1687, 2011.

[26] Centers for Medicare and Medicaid Services. "More Partnerships between Doctors and Hospitals Strengthen Coordinated Care for Medicare Beneficiaries," CMS, 23 December 23, 2013. http://www.cms.gov/Newsroom/MediaReleaseDatabase/Press-Releases/2013-Press-Releases-Items/2013-12-23.html.

[27] Toussaint, J., et al. "How the Pioneer ACO Model Needs to Change: Lessons from its Best-Performing ACO," *Journal of the American Medical Association,* 310(13): 1341-1342, 2013.

[28] Rajkumar, R., et al. "CMS—Engaging Multiple Payers in Payment Report." *Journal of the American Medical Association*, April 21, 2014.

[29] Stanek, Michael. "Quality Measurement to Support Value-Based Purchasing: Aligning Federal and State Efforts," National Academy for State Health Policy, Washington, DC, 2014. http://www.nashp.org/sites/default/files/Quality.Measurement.Support.ValueBasedPurchasing.pdf

[30] Health Information Technology for Economic and Clinical Health (HITECH) Act, Title XIII of Division A and Title IV of Division B of the American Recovery and Reinvestment Act of 2009, Pub. L. No. 111-5, 123 Stat. 226 (Feb. 17, 2009), *codified at* 42 U.S.C. §§300jj *et seq.*; §§17901 *et seq.*

[31] Patient-generated health data are data that are generated by the patient, such as patient satisfaction, health status measures, biometric data, and patient-reported outcomes.

[32] The Federal Government does not aspire to be a repository of health data or health-care data from individuals or private providers. It could, however, through its support for standards-setting and/or other steps, foster and develop public- private partnerships to facilitate exchange and analysis of data, thereby providing meaningful information to consumers and to providers for improvement.

[33] Stage 3 focuses on meaningful use of EHRs for improved outcomes; see: http://www.healthit.gov/providers-professionals/how-attain-meaningful-use

[34] (1) President's Council of Advisors on Science and Technology. *Report to the President- Realizing the Full Potential of Health Information Technology to Improve Healthcare for Americans: The Path Forward.* The White House, December 2010. <http://www.whitehouse.gov/sites/default/files/microsites/ostp/pcast-health-it-report.pdf (1) JASON. "A Robust Health Data Infrastructure," prepared for the Agency for Health Care Research and Quality, AHRQ publication number 14-0041-EF, Rockville, MD, 2014. http://healthit.gov/sites/default/files/ptp13-700hhs_white.pdf

[35] See: http://www.hhs.gov/digitalstrategy/open-data/ or http://healthdata.gov/

[36] Brennan, Niall. "Virtual Research Data Center Offers Secure Timely Access to Data at Lower Cost," *The CMS Blog*, Centers for Medicare and Medicaid Services, November 12, 2013. http://blog.cms.gov/2013/11/12/virtual-research-data-center- offers-secure-timely-access-to-data-at-lower-cost/

[37] See: http://www.medicare.gov/manage-your-health/blue-button/medicare-blue-button.html.

[38] This description was based on personal communication with Richard Newall and draws from: National Research Council. *Principles and Practices for a Federal Statistical Agency*, 5th edition, Washington, DC: National Academies Press, 2013.

[39] Cooperative Extension System offices can be found in every state. See: http://www.csrees.usda.gov/Extension/

[40] See for instance: Gawande, A. "Testing, Testing," *The New Yorker*, December 14, 2009.

[41] Schacht, Wendy. "Manufacturing Extension Partnership Program: An Overview," *Congressional Research Service*. November 20, 2013. https://www.fas.org/sgp/crs/misc/97-104.pdf

[42] See: http://grants.nih.gov/grants/guide/rfa-files/RFA-HS-14-008.html and http://grants.nih.gov/grants/guide/rfa- files/RFA-HS-14-009.html

[43] "Electronic Health Records: Number and Characteristics of Providers Awarded Medicare Incentive Payments for 2011-2012," U.S. Government Accountability Office, October 24, 2013. http://www.gao.gov/products/GAO-14-21R.

[44] Lynch, K., et al. "The Health IT Regional Extension Center Program: Evolution and Lessons for Health Care Transformation," *Health Services Research,* 49(1.2):421-437.

[45] See: http://www.camdenhealth.org/

[46] (1) DeSalvo, Karen. "Community Health Clinics: Bringing Quality Care Closer to New Orleanians," *The New Orleans index at Five: Reviewing Reforms After Hurricane Katrina,* Brookings Institution and Greater New Orleans Community Data Center, August 2010. (2) DeSalvo, K.B., et al. "Community-Based Health Care for 'The City that Care Forgot,'" *Journal of Urban Health,* 82(4):520-523, 2005. (3) DeSalvo, K.B. and S. Kertesz. "Creating a More Resilient Safety Net for Persons with Chronic Disease: Beyond the 'Medical Home,'"*Journal of General Internal Medicine* 22:1377-1379, 2007.

[47] (1) Robert Wood Johnson Foundation. "Coordinating Social and Health Services Improves Care Transition Process," *Promising Practices from the Field,* February 15, 2013. http://www.rwjf.org/en/about-rwjf/newsroom/newsroom- content/2013/02/community-wide-safety-net-improves-care-transitions.html. (2) St. Joseph Health. "Reducing Hospitalizations, Readmissions and Inappropriate Use of Emergency Services," San Francisco. http://sftest.chausa.org/docs/default-source/2013-assembly/c2-reducing-hospitalizations -codron-silva.pdf?sfvrsn=2

[48] (1) Gerhardt, Geoffrey, et al. "Evaluating Whether Changes in Utilization of Hospital Outpatient Services Contributed to Lower Medicare Readmission Rate," *Medicare and Medicaid Research Review* 4:1, 2014. http://www.cms.gov/mmrr/Downloads/MMRR2014_004_01_b03.pdf (2) Barrett, Marguerite, et al. "Conditions With the Largest Number of Adult Hospital Readmissions by Payer," Issue brief No. 172, 2014. http://www.hcup- us.ahrq.gov/reports/statbriefs/sb172-Conditions-Readmissions-Payer.jsp

[49] Hussey, Peter, et al. "From Pilots to Practice: Speeding the Movement of Successful Pilots to Effective Practice," Discussion Paper, Institute of Medicine, April 23, 2013. http://www.iom.edu/~/media/Files/Perspectives- Files/2013/Discussion-Papers/VSRT-VILC-Pilots.pdf

[50] See: http://innovation.cms.gov/initiatives/state-innovations/ and http://innovation.cms.gov/initiatives/CCTP/

[51] (1)"Beacon Community Program," *HealthIT.gov,* n.d. http://www.healthit.gov/policy-researchers-implementers/beacon- community-program (2) Rein, Alison, et al. "Beacon Policy Brief 1.0: The Beacon Community Program, Three Pillars of Pursuit," *HealthIT.gov,* June 3, 2012. http://www.healthit.gov/sites/default/files/pdf/beacon-brief-061912.pdf (3) "The Beacon Community Experience: Illuminating the Path Forward," *HealthIT.gov,* May 22, 2013. http://www.healthit.gov/policy-researchers-implementers/beacon-community-experience-illuminating-path-forward (4) Rein, Alison, et al. "Beacon Policy Brief: Building a Foundation of Electronic Data to Measure and Drive Improvement," *HealthIT.gov,* August 2013. http://www.healthit.gov/sites/default/files/beacon_quality_measurement_brief_final_14aug13.pdf

[52] See: Minnesota Community Measurement at http://mncm.org/

[53] McKethan, A., et al. "An Early Status Report On The Beacon Communities' Plans For Transformation Via Health Information Technology," *Health Affairs* 30(4): 782-788, 2011. Also, see references at footnote 48.

[54] Ibid.

[55] "Hospital Engagement Networks," Centers for Medicare and Medicaid Services. http://partnershipforpatients.cms.gov/about-the-partnership/hospital-engagement-networks/thehospitalengagementnetworks.html

[56] (1) "AHA NOVA Award," *Association for Community Health Improvement*. American Hospital Association, 2013. http://www.aha.org/about/awards/NOVA.shtml (2) "Premier Cares Award: Spotlighting Innovative Programs to Help the Medically Underserved," *Premier, Inc.* https://www.premierinc.com/wps/portal/premierinc/public/aboutpremier/socialresponsibility/caresaward

[57] "Shingo Prize Recipients," *The Shingo Institute*, Utah State University, 2008. http://www.shingoprize.org/shingo-recipients.html

[58] U.S. Department of Commerce. "Baldridge Performance Excellence Program," The National Institute of Standards and Technology, March 25, 2010. http://www.nist.gov/baldrige/

[59] Some institutions, e.g., Arizona State University and Dartmouth College, offer programs in the science of health care delivery. See: https://chs.asu.edu/shcd/academic-programs and http://tdchcds.dartmouth.edu/

[60] See, for example: University of Wisconsin (https://www.xcdsystem.com/shs/proceedings/prof38.html) and Purdue (https://engineering.purdue.edu/IE/ImpactMagazine/ie-impact-magazine2/Purdue_IE%20Impact%20Magazine_Fall%202013.pdf)

[61] See: http://www.ucdmc.ucdavis.edu/nursing/

[62] The diagram and related information were provided by the Oregon Health & Science University (OHSU). http://www.ohsu.edu/xd/

[63] Smith-Bernardin, Shannon, et al. "Safe Sobering: San Francisco's Approach to Chronic Public Inebriation." *Journal of Health Care for the Poor and Underserved (Project Muse )*23, 2012: 265-70. https://www.sfdph.org/dph/files/huh/JHealthCarePoorUnderserved2012 Smith-Bernardin.pdf

[64] (1) Bielaszka-DuVernay, C. "Vermont's Blueprint for medical homes, community health teams, and better health at lower cost," *Health Affairs* (Millwood) 30(3):383-386, 2011. http://hcr.vermont.gov/sites/hcr/files/pdfs/VTBlueprintforHealthAnnualReport2013.pdf (2) Institute of Medicine. "Best Care at Lower Cost: The path to continuously learning health care in America," Washington, DC: National Academies Press, 2012.

[65] President's Council of Advisors on Science and Technology. *Report to the President- Realizing the Full Potential of Health Information Technology to Improve Healthcare for Americans: The Path Forward.* The White House, December 2010. <http://www.whitehouse.gov/sites/default/files/microsites/ostp/pcast-health-it-report.pdf

[66] JASON. "A Robust Health Data Infrastructure," prepared for the Agency for Health Care Research and Quality, AHRQ publication number 14-0041-EF, Rockville, MD, 2014. http://healthit.gov/sites/default/files/ptp13-700hhs_white.pdf

In: A Systems Engineering Approach ...
Editor: Adeline Peaterson

ISBN: 978-1-63321-964-9
© 2014 Nova Science Publishers, Inc.

*Chapter 2*

# RESEARCH AGENDA FOR HEALTHCARE SYSTEMS ENGINEERING[*]

*Ronald L. Rardin*

## EXECUTIVE SUMMARY

Healthcare delivery in the United States is in a crisis of inconsistent and sometimes dismal quality, safety and efficiency, with exploding cost. Paradoxically, while engineering is at the heart of many of the dramatic advances in medical diagnostics and interventions, the engineering that has been done on healthcare delivery processes and operations has had more limited impact, leaving many elements of those delivery systems largely unimproved in half a century. Furthermore, few healthcare professionals are trained to think analytically about delivery systems or even conceive of them as subject to research and engineering.

**Workshop.** This report derives from a workshop of researchers, sponsors, and graduate students held at NSF headquarters in Arlington, Virginia on June 15-16, 2006. Motivated in part by a recent joint study (*Building a Better Delivery System: A New Engineering/Health Care Partnership*, 2005) of the National Academy of Engineers (NAE) and the Institute of Medicine (IOM), the workshop sought to begin the task of envisioning an agenda for Healthcare Systems Engineering (HcSE) research to confront these yawning delivery

---

[*] This is an edited, reformatted and augmented version of a report, primarily sponsored by a National Science Foundation Grant, issued February 2007.

challenges. The Service Enterprise Engineering Program of the Design, Manufacture and Innovation Division at National Science Foundation (NSF) was the principal sponsor. Contributions also came from the National Institutes of Health's (NIH's) National Institute of Biomedical Imaging and Bioengineering (NIBIB) and Purdue University's Regenstrief Center for Healthcare Engineering (RCHE). Although informed by the collection of excellent presentations at the workshop and the associated informal discussions, the opinions expressed in this report are those of the author. Many helpful refinements were also suggested by workshop participants in reviewing early drafts of the report.

**Taxonomies.** The breadth of needed healthcare engineering research is so enormous that it is useful to introduce some organizing taxonomies before turning to specific elements of a research agenda. A first considers the level of the care system to which research is addressed -- whether patient focused on evidence-based choice of interventions for particular cases, population concerned with cost-effective interventions intended for whole populations of patients with like characteristics, team addressed to efforts of frontline care groups, organization concerned with effectiveness and cost of operations and processes within provider facilities, network recognizing the complex mix of organizations and payers who must work together in a decentralizing healthcare delivery system, or environment confronting the regulations, insurance and other payers, consumer and employer interests within which healthcare functions. HcSE research is also classified according to the domain of engineering activity involved – whether technology investigating the tools and components that empower healthcare delivery systems, model-based applying tools of Operations Research, Industrial Engineering, and Operations Management in system design and planning, or practice-based using field trials, survey, and data analysis to improve clinical practice.

**Research Priorities.** The bulk of the report is a systematic presentation of 27 topics of potential research interest organized within the 6 levels of the patient care taxonomy. Research potential for each is evaluated in all 3 of the engineering domains. Those highlighted for priority consideration within the model-based domain of particular interest for this workshop are as follows:

- Treatment Optimization. Formal optimization can often be employed to explicitly or implicitly optimize a measure of treatment success for the patient over the applicable requirements and treatment details. Examples are optimal delivery of radiation therapy for cancer with its plethora of beam angle and intensity choices, and choice of paths of

care for diabetics. The topic has great potential for both new science/methodology innovation and broad healthcare system impact.
- Personalized, Predictive Care. Although its potential is only beginning to even be understood, let alone realized, advances in genomics and proteomics are laying the foundation for transformation in all levels of healthcare by identifying biological markers that both predict health risks and guide the choice of interventions. Modeling and optimization research can have a leading role in how these new protocols for healthcare are delivered if research begins now on how to design, plan and control the new forms of healthcare delivery systems.
- Information Rich and Configurable Operations Management. Operations management research topics centered on the organization level of care have been studied for half a century but remain to realize their full potential. In many cases what is needed is adaptation of fairly well understood methodologies. However, there are special opportunities emerging as widespread information and communications technology finally permeates healthcare delivery facilities. It is also important that more scalable and adjustable forms of operations management models be developed to provide generic tools more easily adapted to widespread application.
- Collaboration Within Networks. Opportunities abound for valuable research targeting collaboration among the many individual provider organizations of modern healthcare networks. The spectrum of attractive topics spans everything from routine provider-to provider handoffs, to emergency response, to home and telehealth, to patient-carequality linked supply chain advances. Two decades of supply chain research in other fields can provide many places to start if sufficient attention is addressed to the performance metrics that make healthcare systems different.
- Large-Scale Delivery System Design. Although not limited to any particular level of care, many of the problems discussed in this report present a similar challenge: optimal design of large-scale delivery systems involving information and communication flows, along with dynamically varying patient demands and provider availabilities, while computing value received and costs incurred to assess performance. Deep and highly valuable research may be possible to produce generic, multi-purpose numerical models that can be adapted to a variety of such healthcare delivery system design tasks.

Important challenges for research in the Human Factors engineering were also highlighted at all levels of care. Patient computer interfaces are a major hurdle to expanded use of home and telehealth care. Electronic medical records and the data entry protocols to support them are an active area of research, but far from successfully resolved. Safety engineering investigations and tools need to be standard in reducing medical errors. Clinical reminders can track cost and warn of danger, but important research is needed on both better technology and user interfaces. Team productivity is critical to effective healthcare, although it is far from well understood, and metrics are largely unavailable to quantify progress.

**Funding the Agenda.** The 2005 NAE/IOM study on a new engineering / healthcare partnership set out a vision for broad new federal investment in academic, engineering-driven research scaled to the dimensions of the critical national need for healthcare delivery transformation in the United States. Unfortunately, that vision is far from realization as this report is written. Instead, HcSE is caught in an inter-agency stalemate, chiefly between the NIH and NSF. NSF is the government's primary home for much of the nation's model-based science and engineering research, but some of its budget-strapped leaders argue that healthcare is NIH's domain, just as energy belongs to the Department of Energy (DOE) and transportation to the Department of Transportation (DOT). However, these analogies are not entirely apt. NIH is indeed the primary home of medical research. But unlike the DOE and DOT cases, systems engineering, especially its model-based healthcare delivery aspects, is not embraced by most parts of NIH and largely incompatible with that agency's organization around medical conditions and demographic groups. Absent major institutional realignment at NIH, NSF appears to be the only federal agency equipped to confront the model-based part of the HcSE challenge.

The limited research which is currently funded has NIBIB and parts of NSF taking the lead in the technology domain of healthcare engineering, NSF with limited help from NIH spearheading model-based research, and primary coverage of the practice-based domain coming from Agency for Healthcare Research and Quality (AHRQ) supported at times by the National Library of Medicine (NLM) and other components of NIH. In the absence of funding appropriate to the research challenge, ways need to be found to maximize the impact of these modest efforts.

- Healthcare Engineering Alliance. Immediate efforts should be made to establish a Healthcare Engineering Alliance among federal sponsors. Modeled after other successful collaborations in manufacturing, nanotechnology and bioengineering, the alliance would hold annual workshops to exchange information on research progress, and coordinate solicitations for grants and contracts. The goal would be to strengthen the working relationships among the agencies that will necessarily be involved in any future acceleration of healthcare engineering research, and to bring more visibility to the field.
- Three-Part Program Leadership. An alliance can provide some degree of strategic leadership in healthcare engineering, but separate focuses of the currently interested agencies will likely sustain for some time. NIBIB should be designated to lead engineering research in the technical domain, NSF should have responsibility for model-based research, and AHRQ should lead on practice-based investigation.
- Partnership Grants. There are numerous challenges where interdisciplinary collaboration among the domains of healthcare engineering is essential. For example, technology advances will have greatest impact if they are utilized in optimally designed delivery systems and planning processes. NSF has experience stimulating collaboration on such interdisciplinary projects with what might be called Partnership Grants. Such grants are joint solicitations from agencies interested in different parts of a problem that are posed with a requirement that all responding teams include one researcher from each domain involved.
- Opportunistic Vigilance. Moving forward to strengthen existing sponsor relationships with collaborative infrastructure cannot relieve either the program managers or the research leaders in healthcare engineering from pursuing opportunities for broader funding. For example, partnerships could be assembled to fit HcSE needs into NSF's huge Cyber Infrastructure program, or to structure one of the Engineering Directorate's Emerging Frontiers in Research and Innovation (EFRI) projects. Also, opportunities for significant funding from agencies of the DOD, state governments, and private foundations need to be further explored.

# 1. INTRODUCTION

## 1.1. The Healthcare Challenge

Healthcare delivery in the United States is in a crisis of inconsistent and sometimes dismal quality, safety, efficiency and access, with exploding cost. It is the largest U.S. industry, currently consuming 15% of the Gross Domestic Product (GDP) and over $6000 per capita. Both these statistics significantly exceed corresponding results for all other developed countries, where healthcare consumes no more than 12% of GDP and $4100 per capita. In addition, U.S. costs are growing at three times inflation because of the rapidly aging population, exploding chronic diseases, and accelerating advances in powerful but expensive medical technology. The resulting financial stress impacts every industry and governments at all levels. At the same time there are serious access shortfalls with over 46 million Americans having no healthcare insurance, many more significantly under-insured, and healthcare constituting the leading cause of personal bankruptcy.

It is paradoxical that while engineering is at the heart of many of the dramatic advances in medical diagnostics and interventions, the engineering that has been done on healthcare delivery processes and operations has had more limited impact, leaving many elements of those delivery systems largely unimproved in half a century. Furthermore, few healthcare professionals are trained to think analytically about delivery systems or even conceive of them as subject to research and engineering. Among the consequences is that lives unnecessarily lost each year in the U.S. due to preventable medical errors are estimated as high as 98,000 and injuries over a million -- higher than losses to auto accidents. An estimated 30-40% of healthcare expenditures go to overuse, underuse, misuse, duplication, system failures, unnecessary repetition, poor communication, and inefficiency. Still, only about half of patients receive best-practice care for their condition. Healthcare is also massively under-invested in information technology, with fewer than 15% of patient records available electronically, and banks spending 4-5 times as much on IT. Coordination and continuity of care are also piecemeal as patients move through a complex of providers, most under separate management with minimal information sharing. The jumble of third party payers funding most of the care, together with distribution of activity across providing institutions and professions, creates perverse economic incentives at every turn.

## 1.2. Healthcare Systems Engineering Workshop

This report derives from a workshop of researchers, sponsors, and graduate students held at NSF headquarters in Arlington, Virginia on June 15-16, 2006. The goal was to begin the task of envisioning an agenda for Healthcare Systems Engineering (HcSE) research to confront the delivery challenges sketched above. Improvements in medical technology, especially IT and communication can provide building blocks. But the systems task is to fashion replicable, predictive models and other tools for designing engineering-integrated systems of personnel, information and communication technologies, and facilities, together with the planning and control regimes that can together transform the safety, cost, quality, and efficiency of healthcare delivery. Leading researchers in the field offered overviews of topic areas, sponsors discussed funding prospects, and breakout groups evolved agendas for future research. The Service Enterprise Engineering Program of the Design, Manufacture and Innovation Division at National Science Foundation (NSF) was the principal sponsor. Contributions also came from the National Institutes of Health's (NIH's) National Institute of Biomedical Imaging and Bioengineering (NIBIB) and Purdue University's Regenstrief Center for Healthcare Engineering (RCHE). (See www.purdue.edu/discoverypark/rche/hcse and the Appendices of to this report for workshop materials and presentations.)

This HcSE workshop was conceived as the counterpart to an earlier one on "Improving Health Care Accessibility Through Point-of-Care Technologies" sponsored primarily by the NIBIB at Crystal City, Virginia on April 11-12, 2006. NSF and other parts of NIH cosponsored. That meeting focused on the supporting technologies of healthcare delivery including biosensors, monitors, imaging and informatics, together with their integration into clinical and telehealth needs. (See www.nibib.nih.gov/publicPage.cfm?pageID=4534)

Although informed by the collection of excellent presentations at both these workshops, and the associated informal discussions, the opinions expressed in this report are those of the author. Many helpful refinements were also suggested by workshop participants in reviewing earlier drafts of the report.

## 1.3. NAE/IOM Study

Both workshops were motivated in part by a recent joint study of the National Academy of Engineers (NAE) and the Institute of Medicine (IOM) entitled *Building a Better Delivery System: A New Engineering/Health Care Partnership* and released in 2005. (Available online at www.iom.edu/CMS/3809/28393.aspx.) The study was funded by NSF, the NIBIB, and the Robert Wood Johnson Foundation.

That NAE/IOM study recommended intensified research on two classes of engineered solutions:

- Delivery facilitating information and communication technology including a comprehensive national health information infrastructure, human-computer interfaces, software for interoperability among vendors, secure and disbursed databases, and microsystems for sensing and monitoring physiological parameters
- Healthcare system engineering modeling, analysis and human factors tools adapted from the systems revolution seen in manufacturing and distribution over recent decades

Both would be energized by a determined effort to cross-educate engineers and healthcare professionals on the value and opportunities for partnership. Another central recommendation of the report is to establish several multidisciplinary centers at institutions of higher learning, funded over 5-10 years at several million dollars per annum and bringing together appropriate fields of engineering, health sciences, management, and social and behavioral sciences. The report describes the centers mission as "(1) to conduct basic and applied research on the systems challenges to health care delivery and on the development and use of systems engineering tools, information /communications technologies, and complementary knowledge from other fields to address them, (2) to demonstrate and diffuse the use of these tools, technologies and knowledge throughout the health care delivery system (technology transfer); and (3) to educate and train a large cadre of current and future health care, engineering, and management professionals and researchers in the science, practices and challenges of systems engineering for health care delivery." Recognizing that funding for such centers would come from a variety of federal agencies, the report also proposes that a lead agency be identified to take the initiative on establishing and sustaining those vital institutions.

## 1.4. Current Sponsors

Unfortunately, none of the federal centers envisioned by the NAE/IOM study has materialized, and no agency has stepped forward to take the lead. Still, there is some support.

- NSF has sustained with a very limited budget the government's only generic research on model-based methods of HcSE. Various other parts of NSF also support research on the cyber-infrastructure and enabling information and control technologies of bioengineering that can empower delivery system advances.
- NIBIB is the lead NIH agency for engineering research on imaging and bioengineering tools that can enable HcSE. However, theirs is one of the smallest budgets of all NIH centers and institutes, and almost no work on actually integrating technologies into delivery processes and operations is supported.
- The National Library of Medicine (NLM) maintains a modest research program on information systems aspects of healthcare delivery.
- Other centers and institutes of the NIH, which are primarily organized around medical conditions or demographic groups, have also sponsored HcSE research in particular circumstances such as National Cancer Institute support of cancer therapy delivery optimization research. However, no single unit leads or coordinates these activities.
- The Agency for Healthcare Research and Quality (AHRQ), which is another part of the Department of Health and Human Services, has taken the lead on practice-based clinical implementation research in healthcare delivery systems. Unfortunately, it too has a budget far below the level required to energize the needed research.
- The Department of Veterans Affairs (VA) has pioneered a number of advances in electronic medical records and patient safety for its own clinical networks. However, it has an explicit policy of doing work internally and limiting support to researchers outside the VA.
- The Department of Defense (DOD) also operates a huge network of healthcare facilities as part of the Military Health System and invests significantly in biomedical research. Prospects for DOD support of academic HcSE research have yet to be explored.

- State departments of health are often interested in particular topics, especially those involving policy issues, access and emergency response.
- Private foundations like the Robert Wood Johnson Foundation have long supported research related to HcSE. However, their attention has increasingly been drawn to national and international policy challenges as opposed to operations, processes and technology for healthcare delivery.

## 1.5. Sources for This Report

The bulk of background information presented in this report is drawn from presentations at the NSF-led workshop in June 2006 and its NIBIB-led counterpart in April 2006, together with material in the NAE/IOM report. Both workshops were introduced in Section 1.2, and full PowerPoint presentations from the June meeting are available online at www.purdue.edu/discoverypark /rche/hcse. Where relevant, these primary sources were supplemented by information in several Institute of Medicine reports: *To Err is Human* (2000), *Crossing the Quality Chasm* (2001), and *Insuring America's Health: Principles and Recommendations* (2004). Some statistics were also drawn from international comparisons of the Organization for Economic Co-operation and Development (OECD, www.oecd.org), and the domestic information in the U.S. Census Bureau's *Income, Poverty, and Health Insurance Coverage in the United States*, www.census.gov/prod/2005pubs /p60-229.pdf. Other useful sources in book form include *Operations Research and Health Care: A Handbook of Methods and Applications*, Kluwer 2004, edited by Margaret Brandeau, Francois Sainfort and William Pierskalla, and the text *Quantitative Methods in Health Care Management: Techniques and Applications*, Jossey-Bass 2005, by Yasar A. Ozcan.

# 2. ORGANIZING TAXONOMIES OF HEALTHCARE ENGINEERING RESEARCH

The breadth of needed healthcare engineering research is so enormous that it is useful to introduce some organizing taxonomies before turning to specific elements of a research agenda. Two are presented here.

## 2.1. Six Levels of Care

One way to categorize healthcare engineering research is to consider the level of the care system to which it is addressed. The NAE/IOM study adapted an earlier 4-level breakdown.

This report adds the refinements of recognizing new Population and provider Network levels to obtain the 6-part scheme depicted in Figure 1.

- **Patient**. At the core of the system is care of individual patients. Research is addressed to evidence-based choice of interventions.
- **Population**. The population level of care addresses cost-effective interventions intended for whole populations of patients with like characteristics.
- **Team**. The team level of analysis focuses on improving the coordinated efforts of the frontline care group, and their collaborations with family and other caregivers.
- **Organization**. Providers work within the component clinical organizations. Research at that level addresses the quality, effectiveness and cost of operations and processes.
- **Network**. An increasingly complex network of collaborating organizations and payers, often with separate goals and ownership, must work together to assure proper care in a decentralizing healthcare delivery system. Network level research addresses methods to align goals and processes for effective collaboration among components of the network.
- **Environment**. All healthcare delivery operations function within an environment of government and professional regulations, insurance and other payers, consumer and employer interests, and more. Research at this level addresses how to better align these policies with effective and cost-efficient healthcare delivery, and how to account for disruptive innovations like the promise of predictive medicine.

## 2.2. Three Engineering Domains

Noting, among other things, the diverse interests of the sponsors sketched in Section 1.4, it will also be useful to classify healthcare engineering research according to the tools and approaches of investigations undertaken.

- **Technology**. One domain investigates the technologies and components that empower improvements in healthcare delivery systems. Sensors, imaging, information technology and communication are central issues, but human-computer interfaces to devices and software are also a major target. The NIBIB is the leading government sponsor in this domain, although others, including NSF and AHRQ, have important roles.

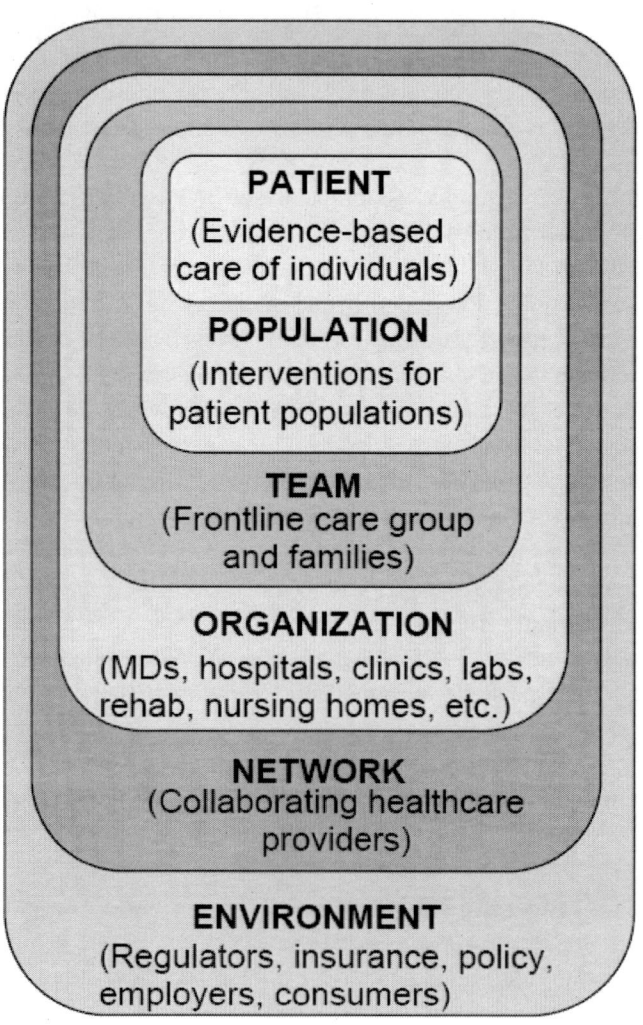

Figure 1. Levels of Care Taxonomy.

- **Model-Based**. Applications of classic tools of Operations Research, Industrial Engineering, and Operations Management center on model-based design, planning and control of healthcare delivery interventions and operations. Included are optimization, simulation, scheduling, Markov systems, games and equilibria, and quality assessment. The target is generic decision systems transferable across many clinical environments. NSF has been the government's main sponsor of this sort of healthcare engineering research.
- **Practice-Based**. The practice-based level of healthcare engineering operates closest to providers and clinics. Drawing on field trials within one or more practices, surveys and data analysis, it seeks to discover process advancements and improved standards for clinical practice. The AHRQ leads government sponsor interest in this domain, although various branches of NIH participate on some topics.

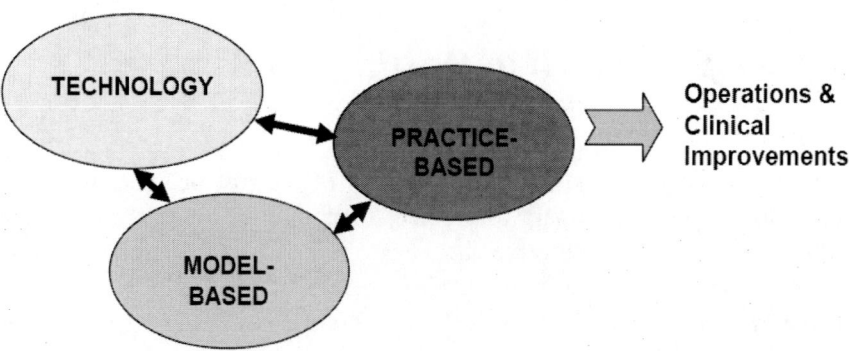

Figure 2. Engineering Domain Taxonomy.

The above figure illustrates how these domains of healthcare engineering combine to produce delivery systems improvements. Technology provides critical building blocks. Model-based analysis integrates personnel, facilities, and technology to improve quality, efficiency and cost. Practice-based investigation refines concepts derived from technology and models in a culture of continuous clinical improvement, while also discovering new challenges for the other two domains. Success often requires intense collaboration among all three.

## 2.3. Essential Role of Practitioner Partnership

This report is about the way forward in Healthcare Systems Engineering (HcSE), and it has been useful to organize the proposed effort according to the six levels of care and the three engineering domains of Sections 2.1 and 2.2. Still, it is important to reaffirm vigorously that almost none of the research to be discussed can be done successfully by engineers and allied technical disciplines alone. No matter how well motivated he/she may be, no engineer can ever understand the challenges in healthcare as well as the professionals who have trained for years and confront the problems every day. Conversely, better understanding and appreciation of HcSE among practitioners is essential for future advances. Success in healthcare engineering research almost always grows out of a solid collaboration with both healthcare professionals and engineering analysts contributing and learning from one another.

## 3. ASSESSMENT OF HEALTHCARE SYSTEMS ENGINEERING TOPICS

Using the taxonomies of Section 2, most of the rest of this report will attempt to provide a summary assessment of numerous topics available for investigation in engineering-driven healthcare research. Although the focus is on research in the narrower topic of Healthcare Systems Engineering, which was the center of the June 2006 workshop, broader issues highlighted in the earlier Point-of-Care workshop in April 2006 and elsewhere are also treated as appropriate. As in all assessments, there are bound to be disagreements among the judgments of different research leaders. Still, the evaluations below are intended to reflect the author's understanding of the rough consensus among those participating in the June HcSE workshop.

Discussions to follow are organized by the six levels of care presented in Section 2.1. To provide a concise summary of each, research topics are enumerated and assessed in a table like the one depicted in Figure 3. The potential of each topic to produce high-value research advances if energetically pursued is evaluated as H=high, M=moderate, or L=low for interest in the Technology, Model-Based, and Practice-Based domains of healthcare engineering described in Section 2.2. Potential is intended to reflect both critical need to find solutions in the problem domain and plausible research paths with great promise. Color/shaded-coding is employed as in Figure 4 for emphasis.

|  | Technology | Model | | Practice |
|---|---|---|---|---|
|  |  | Method | Impact |  |
| Research Topic |  |  |  |  |
|  |  |  |  |  |

Figure 3. Table Format for Concise Assessment.

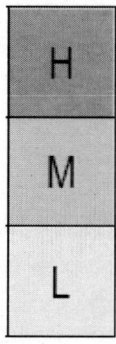

Figure 4. High/Moderate/Low Coding of Topic Potentials.

The model-based domain is the most methodologically and mathematically intense of the three. Thus it is possible to distinguish between the methodology interest of research on a topic versus its impact on the healthcare system. For example, some advances in science/methods will have little short term impact but significantly advance the power of associated tools. Other topics require little new science, but application of currently available methods can produce important healthcare delivery advances. It is for that reason that Method and Impact are scored separately in the Model-Based domain.

## 3.1. Research at the Patient Level of Care

The practice of medicine has always focused on one patient at a time. However, tools of systems engineering have recently demonstrated their potential to assist with clinical decisions by helping stakeholders to investigate the ever more complex array of intervention choices and risks for a given patient. In most cases the analysis is from the point of view of the treating clinical professional, but sometimes tools are intended to help patients decide what risks to take with their own health.

| Research Topic | Technology | Model Method | Model Impact | Practice |
|---|---|---|---|---|
| Practitioner Decision Support | M | M | M | H |
| Patient Decision Support | L | M | M | M |
| Treatment Optimization | M | H | H | M |

*Practitioner Decision Support*

As the variety of conditions to diagnose and interventions to consider grow at an explosive pace, there is an increasing role for computer-based decision aides intended for practitioners. Such research is unlikely to ever replace the judgment of highly trained physicians and nurses, but it can help to assure important considerations are not overlooked. One example is software to assess risks of proposed pharmaceutical prescriptions including drug interactions and allergies. Improvements in technology are important to continuing advances – especially human computer interactions that explore considerations in a user-friendly manner. Model-based tools can enhance the power of such practitioner aides by implementing agreed decision rules and simulating consequences. Still, most of the knowledge base for practitioner decision support comes from practice-based trials. This is especially true of the rapidly growing base of information on customizing care according to genomic and proteomic distinctions among patients.

## Patient Decision Support

In many sorts of medical crises, the patient (and his/her loved ones) needs to take an active role in deciding courses of action. One example is choosing whether to accept an available organ for transplant, taking into account the risks of a poor match now versus likely availability of better choices in the future. Standard methods of interactive decision support can help to structure and inform such weighty decision processes, as well as to facilitate interactions between patient and providers. Technology and model-based aides to such tools are often more readily available and less sophisticated than in the practitioner case. Still, the interactions are certainly informed by insights from practice-based experimentation.

## Treatment Optimization

Once a broad course of action has been selected, formal treatment optimization can often be employed to explicitly or implicitly optimize a measure of treatment success for the patient over the applicable requirements and treatment details. Examples are optimal delivery of radiation therapy for cancer with its plethora of beam angle and intensity choices, and choice of paths of care for diabetics. As with any prediction of human physiological change, there is almost always risk and uncertainty in the decision making. Sometimes it can be ignored, but often it must be explicitly modeled to obtain valid results.

Those developing ever more sophisticated treatment technologies must have at least moderate interest in how they can be optimally employed. Practice-based research also devotes attention to implications for clinical processes and feeds back important insights to optimization formulations. But the heart of this research topic lies in the model-based tools used to accomplish the optimizations. The mathematical challenge and size of the models – especially handling of combinatorial phenomena and uncertainty – makes research in this area likely to yield valuable methodological advances. At the same time the wide variety of health conditions that can be addressed implies both the need for a variety of modeling tools and an enormous potential impact on treatment cost and effectiveness.

## 3.2. Research at the Population Level of Care

Although the ultimate care will be delivered to single patients, population level investigations have long balanced the costs and benefits of interventions being considered for whole classes of individuals. For example, inoculations, laboratory / imaging screening, and similar tools have are core tools of broad public health.

The critical system design issues usually center on what population of individuals are appropriate targets for the intervention, and how it can be delivered to them in the most cost-effective manner. Traditional demographic and condition-based considerations in defining target populations have recently been enriched by growing understanding of bio-chemical markers that differentiate expected responses for different groups.

| Research Topic | Technology | Model | | Practice |
|---|---|---|---|---|
| | | Method | Impact | |
| Patient Screening and Monitoring | H | M | M | H |
| Wellness and Behavior Change | H | M | M | H |
| Personalized, Predictive Care | H | H | H | H |

## *Patient Screening and Monitoring*

Advances in medical technology and results of large population studies yield a continuing stream of opportunities to improve patient outcomes – especially with chronic conditions – by testing physiological parameters. Test-based screening may detect maladies much earlier that waiting for symptoms. Also, monitoring – especially home-based monitoring – can save tremendous cost and keep many patients stable with fewer visits to clinics.

Obviously these methods place a high premium on successful testing and monitoring technologies, and many depend centrally on careful design of patient interactions and processes. There are also important decision problems suitable for model-based research in balancing the costs and health impacts of various mixes of screening and monitoring for particular populations. However, the novelty of tools required and the impact they can have seem moderate compared to those of other domains.

## Wellness and Behavior Change

Results of large population studies also yield a continuing stream of opportunities to improve patient outcomes – especially with chronic conditions – my changing such behavior as eating habits, smoking, and substance abuse. Assessment coupled with behavioral modification counseling can be a lost-cost solution with high health impact.

As pharmaceutical and other tools of mental health come to be employed, and evidence of biological propensities and addiction mechanisms is growing, the potential for technology contributions is rich. There is also high value in careful design of patient interactions and processes. As with screening and monitoring, there are also important decision problems suitable for model-based research in balancing the costs and health impacts of various mixes of interventions. However, the novelty of tools required and the impact they can have again seem moderate compared to those of other domains.

## Personalized, Predictive Care

Advances in genomics and proteomics are laying the foundation for fundamental advances in all levels of healthcare by identifying biological markers that both predict health risks and guide the choice of interventions based on their likelihood of success in populations of patients. That is, the disease-driven, reactive nature of most current healthcare may be transformed over time into a personalized, proactive, wellness-focused delivery system for the $21^{st}$ century.

It is clear that these developments require intensive research in the associated technologies. Furthermore, they are likely to require enormous change in the practice-based processes for collaboration between clinical professionals and their patients. Although it is too early to fully envision, they also seem likely to present model-based planning challenges to structure capacities and flows in any transformed systems, and those will require novel methodologies. Such tools are also likely to have broad health impact because they facilitate the transformation to revolutionary new norms.

## 3.3. Research at the Team Level of Care

Studies at the Team level of care address the small groups of medical professionals, supported by families, who work together on any individual patient case. Information sharing and activity coordination are essential. But they are often hampered by shortages of clinical staff, low morale and work overload, exacerbated by often inadequate supporting information and communication technology.

As demonstrated by the scoring at right, most research in the field requires intense engineering and innovation in technology areas including information and communication systems, and human-computer interaction protocols. Team-level advances are also closely linked with practice-based research on team organization and clinical processes. Model-based research has played a limited role because group processes such as aggregating preferences and avoiding bad outcomes are not well enough understood to support instructive modeling. Impacts that are achieved come mainly from known methodology to find cost-effective mixes of system components.

| Research Topic | Technology | Model | | Practice |
| --- | --- | --- | --- | --- |
| | | Method | Impact | |
| Electronic Medical Records | H | L | M | H |
| Bedside Technology | H | L | M | H |
| Clinical Reminders | H | L | M | H |
| Patient Safety | H | L | M | H |
| Team Productivity | M | M | M | H |

**Electronic Medical Records** are fundamental to tracking what was done to/for a patient and how his/her condition was impacted. Although their availability is growing, in part because of the federal government's National Health Information Infrastructure project, data standards and entry protocols are still subjects of intensive research. Furthermore, it is well established that nurses (and other care providers) spend large fractions of their time foraging for records, test results, and other information required to provide care because the location of such materials is not adequately tracked or recorded in databases.

**Bedside Technology** offers the opportunity to conduct tests and enter data, as well as monitor patient progress without staff running back and forth from other care locations. A major problem is interfacing the variety of new devices being developed into a coordinated records package.

**Clinical Reminders** are designed to warn staff when something should be done or alert them to possible omissions or threats. However, poorly designed human interfaces frequently lead to annoying burdens and information overload for the team.

**Patient Safety** has been a key focus of the healthcare community at least since the notable IOM study *To Err is Human* in 2000 with its alarming estimates of the numbers of patients killed or injured as a result of preventable medical errors. All of the team-level technologies discussed above can contribute to increased patient safety. The various forms of root-cause and Failure Modes and Effects analysis (FMEA) have also become a popular and effective tool for process evaluations to identify, predict and prevent situations inviting dangerous delivery system errors.

**Team Productivity** research investigates how training and other organizational innovations can improve care team effectiveness. Changing roles of different kinds of healthcare professionals must be addressed, as well as how to better incorporate patient friends and loved ones. Exploratory model-based investigations might also help elucidate group processes and evolve useful metrics.

## 3.4. Research at the Organization Level of Care

Research at the health services Organization (e.g. hospital, clinic, physician or other provider) level of care centers around operations management. How should facilities be designed? How should staff and space be used and scheduled? How should patients be scheduled and flowed through the operation? How should the organization's supplies and quality be managed?

These topics are familiar in academic programs in both Industrial Engineering and Operations Management. They have been at the heart of two decades of improvements in the manufacturing and distribution industries.

| Research Topic | Technology | Model Method | Model Impact | Practice |
|---|---|---|---|---|
| Patient Scheduling and Flow | H | H | H | H |
| Facility and Staff Scheduling | M | H | H | M |
| Facilities Location and Design | M | H | H | M |
| Quality Management | M | H | H | M |

There has also been a great deal of healthcare engineering research on these operations topics that spans half a century. Still, its impact on healthcare delivery across the nation has been relatively spotty and modest. Disorganization and lack of coordination, quality gaps, safety risks, resource inefficiencies and growing cost are still the norm in most healthcare operations. As a consequence, clinical professionals have little appreciation for the value systems engineering can bring to operations of their facilities, and little motivation to learn more and seek out engineering partners. Indeed, many regard operations engineering as general management rather than any parallel to the engineering of the medical technologies on which they depend routinely. Some of the explanations include the following:

- The transfer of methods from manufacturing and distribution to healthcare is far from straight-forward, and it is easy to suggest solutions glibly without accounting for differences in the environments. One important distinction is that each patient has unique characteristics and risks, in contrast to the standardization of industrial products on which much of manufacturing operations planning is founded. Another is the sometimes life and death risks to patient's associated with healthcare operations issues that in other contexts involve only marginal changes in service cost.

- The pervasive under-investment in information technology for healthcare operations cripples most quantitative or data-hungry planning and control methodologies. For operations, the issue is less patient medical records than tracking location of patients, providers, and associated resources. Slow progress is being made, but most records continue to be in paper files, with limited use of techniques like bar-coding and radio-frequency identification.
- Perhaps most importantly, the lack of standardization or protocols has meant that most studies on healthcare operations have been one-off investigations directed to a specific application site and building from first principles. Far too few involve generic tools that can easily be adapted to different settings.

This predicament leaves research at the organization level in the dilemma reflected in the scoring matrix above. There is moderate potential for productive research on technology to support operations management, especially information technology to track patients, personnel and resources. Similarly, every subtopic poses practice-based research issues that must be addressed before transforming changes can be effected. As it has in other industries, however, model-based analysis should hold the greatest promise for accelerating change by efficiently exploring wide ranges of alternatives, and investigating their consequences, before any is implemented. In many cases it also depends on coordination of operations management solutions for several topics at the same time. For example, progress on patient flow, or facilities design, may be intricately dependent on innovations in staff scheduling.

## *Patient Scheduling and Flow*

Even though it is among of the longest researched, one of the least fully developed areas of healthcare operations management is scheduling of patient visits and managing patient flow through facilities of the clinic. Traditional systems schedule over long time horizons ignoring or discounting volatility about if and when patients actually show up. Opportunities to distinguish scheduling protocols by non-medical characteristics of patients also are rarely exploited. Furthermore, the share of outpatient care is growing rapidly as hospital stays prove too costly. There, same-day and other dynamic scheduling innovations can have great value. Inside large facilities like hospitals, the issue is tracking patient handoffs among departments and assigning rooms and other resources to deal with dynamic demands. Shared facilities like labs and radiation also complicate flows. All these elements lead to important opportunities for technology advances in tracking, and in configurable, dynamic, model-based planning and control innovations, as well as important improvements in clinical processes to exploit better planning.

## *Facilities and Staff Scheduling*

Scheduling of clinical staff such as nurse work shifts, and of critical facilities like operating rooms, are some of the most researched topics in healthcare operations management. Still, much current scheduling is manual, and the challenges of diverse shifts and staffing level requirements are, if anything, growing more complex. As noted earlier, a principal requirement is wider implementation of what is known. Still, there remain opportunities for innovative technology, processes, and configurable modeling tools to address dynamic changes in demands through time and even more complex staffing norms.

## *Facilities Location and Design*

Aging of both the patient population and the large generation of hospitals built in the Hill-Burton era of the 1950's and 1960's has produced a boom in hospital and other clinic construction. This offers a real opportunity for high-impact healthcare engineering addressed to facilities location and design. Model-based tools are available from other domains for the locations questions, but internal design offers many opportunities for innovation. New hospitals must be equipped for ever growing information and bedside technology, and spaces must be flexible enough to respond to variability in demand, often with a smaller number of beds than in older facilities.

## *Quality Management*

Tracking and controlling the quality of medical facility operations is obviously of the highest importance to improvement in healthcare delivery. As on other topics, there is great scope for adapting methods developed for similar challenges in other industries such as Six Sigma. However, all those tools must be modified to confront a fundamental difference in controlling healthcare operations: each patient has different attributes, different risks, and different prospects. Research on risk-adjusted methods and measures remains to be fully explored.

## 3.5. Research at the Network Level of Care

This report has added a Network level of care between individual health providers and the broad environment because of the increasing decentralization of healthcare operations across a variety of different types of providers. Besides hospitals and physicians working alone or in small partnerships, there are ambulatory clinics, diagnostic centers, nursing homes, rehab facilities, pharmacists, home care services, several forms of telecare, and third-party payers. Patients move back and forth among all these providers with their separate goals and management, and minimal information sharing. Indeed, the current state of affairs has been described as a non-system or a cottage industry.

| Research Topic | Technology | Model | | Practice |
| --- | --- | --- | --- | --- |
| | | Method | Impact | |
| Secure Information Sharing | H | M | M | H |
| Collaborative Operations | L | H | H | M |
| Emergency Collaboration | M | H | H | H |
| Supply Chain Management | M | H | H | M |
| Home Care | H | H | H | H |
| Provider-to-Provider Telehealth | H | L | M | H |
| Perverse Incentives | L | H | H | M |

### *Secure Information Sharing*

If patient records are to a shared among providers, with patients and their families, and even with medical informatics researchers, protocols must be developed to protect privacy while at the same time allowing quick and user-friendly data entry and retrieval. Although secure communication has been an active topic of research in computer science for many years, protocols and standards remain far from fully mature. Also, confidentiality in healthcare extends well beyond data encryption. This is especially true when patient data is being interrogated as part of medical research or field trials. Sensitive personal data has to be protected while allowing researchers to attribute causes of disparities seen in outcomes. Research on healthcare sharing and privacy is also intertwined with practice-based development of processes, as well as design of novel human-computer interfaces. Model-based research can contribute in choosing minimum cost and high reliability combinations of available components, but its role is likely to be secondary.

*Collaborative Operations*

Even after adequate information sharing systems have been devised, there will remain a plethora of problems in coordinating the treatment of patients as they flow through providers with different management, cost incentives, and purposes. Continuity of care is at risk if providers do not properly manage transfers, and in/out flows of one provider can severely impact the capacity management decisions of another. Perhaps most influential are payment and reimbursement structures and how they incentivize or discourage different care protocols. Technology challenges in collaboration other than through IT are relatively modest, but there remain many process targets for practice-based research. Model-based analyses of healthcare collaboration issues are currently rare, but two intense decades of related research in manufacturing supply chains and out-sourced operations is waiting to be adapted to healthcare issues. That work has established through game/equilibrium modeling and computer simulations how value-sharing and incentive arrangements can be structured that align the objectives and yield economic gain for all collaborators.

*Emergency Collaboration*

Although related, a host of new collaboration issues arise when the healthcare system in a region is confronted by a disease, terrorism, or natural emergency. The new elements are communication technologies for command and control, and protocols for sharing resources and managing their allocation. Besides the collaborative decision-making tools appropriate for regular operations, high-impact model-based research should also evaluate how to place and equip providers for resiliency and rapid reconfigurability in the face of emergencies. It is particularly timely to investigate these issues in the context of the current healthcare facility building boom, and the national emphasis on pandemic and terror threats.

## *Supply Chain Management*

Medical facilities consume vast quantities of sometimes high-value and perishable supplies and equipment. This includes everything for cleaning materials, to pharmaceuticals, to electronics, to implantable devices and joints. The network of manufacturers, group purchasing organizations, third-party logistics firms, and providers themselves that manages these supplies is composed of different players than those of the provider delivery networks discussed so far, but it is subject to all the same requirements for collaboration and alignment of objectives. Furthermore, the rich technologies and lessons of supply chain management research in manufacturing over the past two decades, such as lean and just-in-time procurement, and postponement to facilitate product customization, remain to be broadly mined in many aspects of healthcare. There appears to be substantial opportunity for cost savings while improving availability of materials when they are needed, both of which will make direct contributions to quality and safety of healthcare. However, such advances await important model/method development to adapt tools from other domains to healthcare where performance metrics emphasize quality and safety of patient care above other considerations. In particular, extra attention to risk management may also be critical in model-based approaches because the consequences of stock outs are potentially much greater when human health is involved.

## *Home Care*

Provider outreach and telehealth links in the home span a wide range of systems from home patient visits by nurses, to telecom followup on patients by providers, to remote monitoring of patient physiological parameters. Use of these systems is growing, and they represent a potential opportunity to improve access for rural and other underserved populations, yield significant cost savings, and improve patient satisfaction. However, more widespread application awaits healthcare engineering research of nearly every type. User friendly patient interfaces for persons with little computer literacy are a critical human factors design challenge. Practice-based research is needed on nearly every form of home telehealth to maximize quality and effectiveness of services delivered, while reducing costs. So much is to be decided about the best way to locate facilities, allocate and route staff, provide reliable computer links, and other elements of system design that there should also be a strong opportunity for novel new models that challenge the limits of current model-based methodology.

### *Provider to Provider Telehealth*

Use of telemedicine among spatially distributed providers is another growing dimension of telehealth. It extends from (sometimes global) consultations with specialists not available at the primary care site to remotely controlled robotic procedures. As with the home version of telehealth, they represent a potential opportunity to improve access for rural and other underserved populations, and to reap significant cost savings. Also like the home case, human-computer interfaces are central research issues. But that challenge is somewhat less daunting because those interacting are highly trained medical professionals. On the other hand secure communication of patient documents and images are of greater importance, and advances in practice-based protocols are critical. With the scale of communication networks much smaller and less diverse than those for home care, model-based analysis is likely to center on application of known network-design tools.

### *Perverse Incentives*

An important special set of issues in network collaboration arises when competing incentives for different providers have the effect of risking patient health and/or inflating overall system costs. For example, monitoring patients in their homes may reduce the need for return visits to hospitals. The result is increased revenue to telehealth providers, significantly reduced treatment cost, and improved patient satisfaction, but there may be a significant loss of revenue for hospitals. Again, the model-based tools of supply chains and distributed operations should be adaptable to quantifying effects and structuring collaborative arrangements that align interests with overall system and patient health objectives.

## 3.6. Research at the Environment Level of Care

Research at the Environment level of care quickly touches the controversies about national healthcare policy that have challenged decision makers for at least the last 60 years. Goals are to realign incentives – especially financial ones – to avoid perverse behavior seen in the present system.

# Research Agenda for Healthcare Systems Engineering 93

| Research Topic | Technology | Model Method | Model Impact | Practice |
|---|---|---|---|---|
| Capitation vs. Pay for Procedures | L | M | M | H |
| Pay for Performance | L | M | M | H |
| Consumer-Based Healthcare | L | M | M | H |
| Cross Subsidization | L | M | M | H |
| Predictive Care Transformation | H | H | H | H |

In most cases technology is not a major issue. Instead decisions are informed mostly by high-impact, practice-based studies and demonstration projects across samples of providers. Model-based research – here mostly economic modeling – can do preliminary investigations of possible solutions and estimate their consequences before they receive more field testing. It can also estimate the broad consequences of extending an apparently successful test to wide national implementation.

## *Capitation vs. Pay for Procedures*

One of the most enduring controversies in healthcare policy is whether insurance payers should reimburse providers on a per-patient or capitation basis versus paying for particular procedures as they may be medically indicated. Moving from one to the other clearly has dramatic impacts on the incentives and risks of the payers and the patient. For example, capitation can present providers with enormous financial risk to cases where unexpected but expensive medical complications arise. Conversely, payments for procedures create a bias away from holistic internal medicine in favor of specialists who do expensive interventions.

## *Pay for Performance*

An incentive strategy of more recent origin, termed Pay for Performance, seeks to reward providers based on their history of quality. Reimbursement is fractionally increased for those with good records and/or decreased for those with weaker performance. Development of valid quality measures on which to base such incentives is a challenging topic of research.

## *Consumer-Based Healthcare*

As healthcare costs to employers and government payers accelerate, there is increasing interest in reimbursement schemes where the consumer plays a more active role in treatment choices, and bears more of the financial risk. The intent is to create competitive market pressures for consumers to take their healthcare needs to providers they believe offer the best balance of service quality and price. Such systems also offer the promise of increased leverage to achieve patient-centered care, improved patient compliance with care regimes, and greater patient attention to prevention and wellness as increased responsibility for their care falls on the patient. Major hurdles are that few patients are knowledgeable enough about what healthcare they need to make informed decisions, and fewer still know what providers can offer it, and how they should be compared. Thus, movement to a more consumer-based form of healthcare will require intensive research on how to collect and communicate appropriate care and provider performance data.

## *Cross Subsidization*

The US healthcare market can be subdivided into approximately 27% who have healthcare provided by government, 15% with no healthcare insurance at all, and most of the remainder funded by private employers. Ethical standards and federal law require that providers serve all these populations regardless of the patient's ability to pay. But substantial pressure on reimbursement rates by government payers, and little or no collections from the uninsured, have left providers balancing revenues and costs by increasing charges for privately funded treatment. This cross subsidization is a major and growing burden for private employers that needs to be better quantified and understood if solutions are to be found.

## *Predictive Care Transformation*

The nascent revolution in personalized, predictive care has already been introduced under Population care in Section 3.2. Advances in genomics and proteomics are laying the foundation for fundamental advances in all levels of healthcare by identifying biological markers that both predict health risks and guide the choice of interventions based on their likelihood of success with individual patients. That is, the disease-driven, reactive nature of current healthcare may be transformed over time into a personalized, proactive, wellness-focused delivery system for the 21$^{st}$ century.

Besides offering new challenges in the provision of care -- including technology, practice protocols, and related planning modeling tools -- the prospect of a predictive care transformation will have enormous impact for policy makers at all levels. New institutions and infrastructures will likely be required, and payment/incentives systems are bound to be adjusted. Although it is too early to fully envision, these seem likely to present model-based planning challenges to structure capacities and flows in transformed systems, and those will require novel methodologies with broad health impact.

## 4. BROAD CONCLUSIONS AND RECOMMENDATIONS

The detailed discussions of Sections 3.1-3.6 offer a host of conclusions about the potential for research on numerous healthcare engineering topics. This final section of the report addresses two broader issues: what topics in the Healthcare Systems Engineering (HcSE) scope of this workshop deserve research priority, and how a partnership among funding agencies can begin addressing the stalemate preventing realization of the academic healthcare engineering vision in the NAE/IOM study.

### 4.1. Priorities for Model-Based Healthcare Systems Research

Some high potential topics discussed in Section 3 that are most central to the model-based systems engineering part of HcSE deserve priority support – likely under NSF funding leadership.

- **Treatment Optimization**. Formal optimization can often be employed to explicitly or implicitly optimize a measure of treatment success for the patient over the applicable requirements and treatment details. This category of research has great potential for both new science/methodology and broad system impact because the approach is useful in so many different environments. Each requires different modeling and optimization tools, and each offers a different set of implementation challenges.
- **Personalized, Predictive Care**. Although its potential is only beginning to even be understood, let alone realized, a revolution in

personalized, proactive healthcare seems certain to burst out within the next generation. Modeling and optimization research can have a leading role in how these new protocols for healthcare are delivered if research begins now on how to design, plan and control the new forms of healthcare delivery systems.

- **Information Rich and Configurable Operations Management.** Operations management research topics centered on the organization level of care have been studied for half a century but remain to realize their full potential. In many cases what is needed is adaptation of fairly well understood methodologies. However, there are special opportunities emerging as widespread information and communications technology finally permeates healthcare delivery facilities. Information-rich forms of delivery systems management supported by readily available data on patient traffic and provider resource loading will both catalyze new methods and offer tremendous system impact. It is also important that more scalable and adjustable forms of operations management models be developed to provide generic tools more easily adapted to widespread application. This includes refining patient scheduling and flow planning tools to address particular patient populations and newer, outpatient-oriented modes of care.
- **Collaboration Within Networks.** Opportunities abound for valuable research targeting collaboration among the many individual provider organizations of modern healthcare networks. As information systems and sharing become more widespread, new design, planning and control tools will be needed to avoid duplication and perverse incentives, while maintaining high quality continuity of care and providing value to all participants. The spectrum of attractive topics spans everything from routine provider-to-provider handoffs, to emergency response, to home and telehealth, to patient-care-quality linked supply chain advances. Two decades of supply chain research in other fields can provide many places to start if sufficient attention is addressed to the performance metrics that make healthcare systems different.
- **Large-Scale Delivery System Design.** Although not limited to any particular level of care, many of the problems discussed in Section 3 present a similar challenge: optimal design of large-scale delivery systems involving information and communication flows, along with dynamically varying patient demands and provider availabilities,

while analyzing value received and costs incurred to assess performance. Monte Carlo computer simulations can be used for some such tasks, but their development cost is high, and each is closely linked to a particular setting. Deep and highly valuable research may be possible to produce generic, multi-purpose numerical models that can be adapted to a variety of healthcare delivery system design tasks.

## 4.2. Priorities for Human Factors Healthcare Delivery Research

The focus of the June Workshop which stimulated this report is the NSF-related model-base topics highlighted in Section 4.1. Still, Section 3 notes research needs in the Human Factors field at almost every level of care, and across both the technology and the practice-based engineering domains. Although not likely to be concerns for NSF, the following topics seen to warrant high priority with other sponsors:

- **Patient Computer Interfaces**. Home and telehealth care offer tremendous opportunities for reducing costs, improving healthcare quality, expanding access, and achieving greater patient satisfaction. But progress is critically hindered by the challenge of having older patients, and ones with limited computer literacy, easily interface with the internet and telecommunication. Accelerated research on both new devices and interchange protocols is urgent.
- **Data Entry and Display for Electronic Medical Records**. Although the topic has received great attention for more than a decade, the challenge of efficient and reliable data entry and retrieval for electronic medical records systems remains far from fully resolved. How should providers log their treatment and judgments about patients in accessible ways? How can we avoid replacing formal clerical entry processes for data collection by much more expensive and equally burdensome entry by clinical professionals?
- **Safety Engineering to Avoid Medical Errors.** Application of safety engineering methods developed in the airline and nuclear industries has proved highly valuable in finding safety weaknesses in proposed processes and identifying the root cause of medical errors. Given the critical importance of reducing unnecessary and often costly medical errors, continued investment in research on process and resilient

computerized alert systems that extend the power of existing tools is essential.
- **Point of Care Clinical Reminders.** An important element of human factors research should focus on the computerized systems that support point of care healthcare delivery by communicating progress and warning about dangerous trends. There is a great deal of this sort of technology presently in use or coming, but a balance has not been achieved in the data entry and information load team members are expected to bear in order for the alerts to be effective.
- **Team Productivity.** At every stage, from delicate surgery to home and rural care, healthcare is a team effort. Research on how to train professionals and shape their roles in enhance productivity is important to improving quality and reducing costs and errors.

An important element is development of metrics to quantify productivity, especially as it relates to outcomes of care.

## 4.3. Funding the Agenda

As briefly discussed in Sections 1.3, the 2005 NAE/IOM study on a new engineering / healthcare partnership set out a vision for broad new federal investment in academic, engineering-driven research. The effort was to be scaled to the dimensions of the critical national need for healthcare delivery transformation, with one federal agency assuming the lead as a critical step to future progress.

Unfortunately, the review in Section 1.4 highlights how far that vision is from realization as this report is written. Instead, HcSE is caught in an inter-agency stalemate, mainly between NIH and NSF. NSF is the government's primary home for much of the nation's model-based science and engineering research, but some of its budget-strapped leaders argue that healthcare is NIH's domain, just as energy belongs to DOE and transportation to DOT. However, these analogies are not entirely apt. NIH is indeed the primary home of medical research. But unlike the DOE and DOT cases, systems engineering, especially its model-based healthcare delivery aspects, is not embraced by most parts of NIH and largely incompatible with that agency's organization around medical conditions and demographic groups. Absent major institutional realignment at NIH, NSF is the only federal agency equipped to confront the model-based part of the HcSE challenge.

One major challenge of this workshop and report is to find a way forward that begins to deal with this crippling funding stalemate. Relevant research is underway on a limited scale (see Section 1.4), with NIBIB and parts of NSF taking the lead in the technology domain of healthcare engineering, NSF with help from NIH spearheading model-based research, and primary coverage of the practice-based domain coming from AHRQ supported at times by the NLM and other components of NIH. This predicament is far less than acceptable. But it may be all there is to work with for some time, and ways need to be found to maximize its impact.

- **Healthcare Engineering Alliance**. Immediate efforts should be made to establish a Healthcare Engineering Alliance among federal sponsors. Modeled after other successful collaborations in manufacturing, nanotechnology and bioengineering, the alliance would hold annual workshops to exchange information on research progress, and coordinate solicitations for grants and contracts. The goal would be to strengthen the working relationships among the agencies that will necessarily be involved in any future acceleration of healthcare engineering research, and to bring more visibility to the field.
- **Three-Part Program Leadership**. An alliance can provide some degree of strategic leadership in healthcare engineering, but separate focuses of the currently interested agencies will likely sustain for some time. NIBIB should be designated to lead engineering research in the technical domain, NSF should have responsibility for model-based research, and AHRQ should lead on practice-based investigation. None of these three would be the only sponsor in their designated domain, but they should be responsible for taking the lead.
- **Partnership Grants**. There are numerous challenges where interdisciplinary collaboration among the domains of healthcare engineering is essential. For example, technology advances will have greatest impact if they are utilized in optimally designed delivery systems and planning tools. Similarly, economic insights from model-based research can suggest critical technology needs to open the way for high-value gains.

NSF has experience stimulating collaboration on such interdisciplinary projects with various parts of the NIH, the Environmental Protection Agency, the Department of Transportation, the National Aeronautics and Space Administration, and others. An effective tool for stimulating collaboration on such interdisciplinary projects has been what might be called Partnership Grants. Such grants are joint solicitations from agencies interested in different parts of a problem that are posed with a requirement that all responding teams include one researcher from each domain involved. For example the solicitation might call for at least one researcher interested in physiological sensors to collaborate with another interested in optimal facility layout in evolving a new bedside approach to care.

It is undeniably true that all such collaborations are awkward and burdensome for the agencies involved, especially in how they align their peer review processes. But the benefits of truly interdisciplinary research in healthcare engineering and of community building for the whole research effort should outweigh such difficulties.

- **Opportunistic Vigilance.** Moving forward to strengthen existing sponsor relationships with collaborative infrastructure cannot relieve either the program managers or the research leaders in healthcare engineering from pursuing opportunities for broader funding. For example, partnerships could be assembled to fit HcSE needs into NSF's huge Cyber Infrastructure program, or to structure one of the Engineering Directorate's Emerging Frontiers in Research and Innovation (EFRI) projects. Also, opportunities for significant funding from agencies of the DOD, state governments, and private foundations need to be further explored.

# INDEX

## #

21st century, 83, 95

## A

abuse, 41
access, 1, 2, 4, 5, 14, 23, 25, 38, 46, 47, 48, 49, 50, 52, 62, 70, 74, 91, 92, 97
accountability, 16
accounting, 86
accreditation, 4, 31, 32
adaptation, 27, 67, 96
administrators, 4, 25, 37
adults, 28, 42
advancements, 77
adverse event, 48, 60
age, 42
agencies, 27, 32, 45, 47, 48, 52, 69, 72, 95, 99, 100
aggregation, 47
aging population, 70
Air Force, 54
alcohol abuse, 41
ALS, 21
American Recovery and Reinvestment Act, 6, 44, 60, 62
American Recovery and Reinvestment Act of 2009, 62
appetite, 34

appointments, 6, 28, 29
assessment, 4, 31, 32, 77, 78
authority, 52
aviation, vii
awareness, 4, 25, 34

## B

background information, 74
bandwidth, 12
bankruptcy, 70
banks, 70
barriers, 2, 13, 14, 32
base, 23, 80, 94, 97
behavioral sciences, 72
benchmarking, 16, 17
benchmarks, 52
beneficiaries, 16, 23, 24, 60
benefits, 47, 48, 49, 51, 81, 100
bias, 93
biological markers, 67, 83, 94
biosensors, 71
blood, 42
bloodstream, 61
breakdown, 75
building blocks, 71, 77
burnout, 10
business processes, 18
businesses, 1, 6, 22, 38

## C

cancer, 66, 73, 81
care model, 6, 20
caregivers, 75
catheter, 61
CDC, 21, 31, 44, 47, 48
Census, 21, 74
certification, 36
challenges, vii, 4, 8, 10, 12, 13, 22, 24, 25, 28, 34, 38, 40, 48, 50, 52, 66, 68, 69, 71, 72, 74, 77, 78, 83, 88, 90, 95, 99
chemical, 82
Chief of Staff, 54
children, 41
chronic diseases, 12, 70
City, 41, 63, 71
classes, 35, 72, 82
cleaning, 91
coding, 79, 87
collaboration, vii, 4, 21, 25, 35, 36, 41, 62, 67, 69, 75, 77, 78, 83, 90, 91, 92, 96, 99
collaborative approaches, 33
commercial, 3, 7, 17
communication, 33, 35, 36, 67, 70, 71, 72, 76, 84, 90, 92, 96
communication systems, 84
communication technologies, 71, 90
communities, 2, 4, 11, 14, 25, 27, 28, 30, 31, 37, 38
community, vii, 2, 3, 4, 8, 10, 11, 12, 13, 16, 19, 24, 25, 27, 28, 29, 30, 31, 32, 34, 41, 46, 49, 51, 63, 64, 85, 100
complexity, 9, 43
compliance, 94
complications, 15, 93
computer, 68, 72, 76, 80, 84, 90, 91, 92, 97
computer simulations, 90, 97
computing, 67
concise, 79
confidentiality, 90
congress, 46
consensus, 78
consolidation, 13
construction, 88
consulting, 44
consumers, 24, 62, 94
controversies, 92, 93
coordination, 10, 27, 43, 45, 83, 86, 87
cost, 4, 7, 8, 12, 15, 16, 23, 25, 27, 43, 52, 60, 62, 64, 65, 66, 68, 70, 71, 75, 77, 81, 82, 83, 84, 86, 90, 91, 92, 97
cost saving, 91, 92
counseling, 83
covering, 23, 24
crises, 81
culture, 13, 77
curricula, 4, 37
curriculum, 35, 36
cycles, 12, 34

## D

danger, 68
data analysis, 48, 52, 66, 77
data collection, 46, 53, 97
data mining, 51
data set, 17, 20, 52, 53
decentralization, 89
decision makers, 92
Department of Commerce, 4, 25, 27, 35
Department of Defense, 23, 44, 48, 73
Department of Energy, 22, 44, 68
Department of Health and Human Services, 21, 44, 47, 60, 73
Department of Transportation, 68, 99
detection, 51
developed countries, 70
diabetes, 11, 30
diffusion, 33
diffusion group, 33
discharges, 12
diseases, 6
distribution, 13, 70, 72, 85, 86
diversity, 7, 8, 14, 28, 49, 50
DOT, 68, 98
drug interaction, 80

## E

economic incentives, 70
education, 7, 12, 26, 34, 35, 36, 37
emergency, 12, 28, 29, 41, 42, 67, 74, 90, 96
emergency response, 42, 67, 74, 96
employers, 3, 17, 32, 52, 62, 94
encryption, 90
energy, 22, 68, 98
entrepreneurship, 49, 52
environment(s), vii, 6, 7, 27, 35, 42, 43, 66, 75, 77, 86, 89, 95
environmental influences, 42
Environmental Protection Agency, 99
equilibrium, 90
equipment, 8, 91
evidence, 6, 10, 11, 12, 23, 25, 26, 28, 32, 35, 42, 66, 75, 83
evidence-based program, 28
expenditures, 41, 70
expertise, 7, 18, 45
exports, 22

## F

false alarms, 8
families, 1, 2, 6, 38, 83, 89
farmers, 25
federal agency, 68, 98
Federal Government, 18, 62, 84
federal law, 94
field trials, 66, 77, 90
financial, 33, 70, 92, 93, 94
flexibility, 51
flights, 7
food, 29
Food and Drug Administration (FDA), 21, 44, 47, 48
force, 47
foundations, 32, 33, 69, 74, 100
fraud, 51
funding, vii, 4, 30, 37, 41, 68, 69, 70, 71, 72, 95, 99, 100

## G

GAO, 44, 63
GDP, 70
genomics, 51, 67, 83, 94
governance, 31, 52
governments, 69, 70, 100
graduate students, 35, 65, 71
grant programs, 4, 37
grants, 29, 30, 63, 69, 99, 100
grassroots, 32
Gross Domestic Product, 70
group processes, 84, 85
guidance, 26
guidelines, 18, 20, 31

## H

harmonization, 45, 51
Hawaii, 61
hazardous substances, 21
Health and Human Services, 3, 17, 19, 24, 27, 32, 35, 37, 60
health care, vii, 1, 2, 4, 6, 7, 9, 10, 11, 12, 13, 14, 15, 16, 18, 23, 26, 27, 33, 34, 35, 37, 38, 39, 41, 42, 43, 48, 49, 53, 60, 61, 64, 72
health care costs, 48
health care system, vii, 4, 26, 49, 61
health condition, 81
health information, 3, 12, 17, 18, 19, 20, 31, 41, 45, 47, 48, 49, 52, 72
health insurance, 5
health practitioners, 37
health problems, 12
health risks, 67, 83, 94
health services, 10, 85
health status, 18, 28, 31, 62
health-care organizations, vii, 1, 7, 10, 16, 18, 27, 31, 34, 37, 38
heart attack, 11
heart disease, 11, 30
HHS, 3, 4, 17, 19, 20, 21, 22, 24, 25, 32, 37, 44, 45, 48, 49, 52, 53

high blood pressure, 11
hiring, 52
history, 93
home care services, 89
homes, 41, 64, 92
host, 90, 95
housing, 29
hub, 29
human, 7, 9, 42, 43, 72, 76, 80, 81, 84, 85, 90, 91, 92, 98
human health, 91
Hurricane Katrina, 29, 63
hypertension, 12, 61

# I

identification, 48, 87
identity, 50
images, 92
imports, 22
improvements, 12, 16, 39, 76, 77, 85, 88
incidence, 60
income, 28
independence, 22
indexing, 46, 51
individuals, 3, 17, 29, 41, 48, 62, 82
industries, 1, 7, 38, 85, 87, 88, 97
industry, 22, 70, 89
inefficiency, 70
infection, 11
inflation, 70
information sharing, 70, 89, 90
information technology, 3, 46, 70, 76, 87
infrastructure, vii, 2, 3, 12, 14, 18, 19, 20, 29, 30, 38, 45, 47, 48, 49, 50, 51, 52, 69, 72, 73, 100
injuries, 70
institutions, 20, 35, 64, 70, 72, 95
integration, 4, 25, 46, 49, 71
intelligence, 53
interface, 51, 97
internship, 35
interoperability, 18, 20, 46, 48, 49, 50, 51, 72
intervention, 40, 61, 80, 82

investment(s), 52, 53, 68, 87, 97, 98
issues, 22, 28, 37, 43, 48, 76, 78, 82, 86, 87, 90, 92, 95

# J

joints, 91

# L

landscape, 22
languages, 28
lead, 1, 6, 24, 36, 49, 68, 69, 72, 73, 85, 87, 98, 99
leadership, 3, 4, 13, 24, 25, 34, 36, 37, 51, 69, 95, 99
learning, 4, 18, 33, 37, 64, 72, 78
legislation, 22
lens, 14
life cycle, 39, 43
lifelong learning, 35
literacy, 91, 97
living conditions, 28
local employers, 16
local government, 10
localization, 26
logistics, 43, 91
Louisiana, 29

# M

management, vii, 7, 9, 10, 26, 34, 42, 53, 67, 70, 72, 85, 86, 87, 88, 89, 90, 91, 96
manufacturing, vii, 7, 25, 42, 69, 72, 85, 86, 90, 91, 99
manufacturing companies, 25
mapping, 9, 42, 45
materials, 40, 43, 71, 85, 91
matrix, 87
matter, 16, 78
measurement(s), 3, 16, 17, 34, 43, 63
media, 61, 63
Medicaid, 3, 6, 17, 18, 20, 21, 26, 32, 33, 41, 44, 46, 54, 57, 62, 63

medical, 2, 6, 11, 13, 15, 20, 28, 29, 31, 36, 37, 41, 48, 49, 51, 60, 61, 64, 65, 68, 70, 71, 73, 81, 82, 83, 85, 86, 87, 88, 89, 92, 93, 97, 98
medical care, 60
Medicare, 3, 6, 16, 17, 18, 20, 21, 23, 24, 26, 28, 30, 32, 33, 41, 44, 46, 47, 52, 54, 57, 60, 62, 63
medication, 28
medicine, 17, 75, 80, 93
mental health, 29, 83
methodology, 67, 79, 84, 92, 95
Microsoft, 58
mission, 36, 72
misuse, 47, 70
models, 2, 10, 13, 16, 26, 29, 30, 67, 71, 77, 81, 92, 96, 97
modernization, 46, 47
modules, 36
morale, 83
mortality, 9, 11, 61
mortality rate, 9, 61
motivation, 86
multiple factors, 17, 29

## N

nanotechnology, 69, 99
National Aeronautics and Space Administration, 99
National Health and Nutrition Examination Survey, 21
National Health Information Infrastructure, 84
National Institutes of Health, 18, 22, 44, 66, 71
National Research Council, 62
National Survey, 21, 22
natural disaster, 29
negotiating, 16
New England, 60, 61
next generation, 96
NRC, 46
nurses, 4, 14, 36, 37, 80, 84, 91
nursing, 35, 36, 41, 47, 64, 89

nursing home, 47, 89

## O

obesity, 30
objectivity, 22
OECD, 74
Office of Management and Budget, 22, 45
OMB, 22, 45
operations, vii, 2, 7, 8, 9, 11, 15, 25, 30, 32, 34, 38, 65, 66, 67, 70, 73, 74, 75, 77, 85, 86, 87, 88, 89, 90, 92, 96
opportunities, 4, 6, 19, 25, 28, 34, 35, 49, 67, 69, 72, 82, 83, 88, 96, 97, 100
optimism, 35
optimization, vii, 43, 66, 67, 73, 77, 81, 95, 96
optimization method, 43
organ, 81
organizational culture, 12
organizational learning, 42
organize, 78
outpatient, 87, 96
outreach, 91
overproduction, 40
ownership, 75

## P

pain, 15
parallel, 46, 86
parents, 6
participants, 66, 71, 96
patient care, 20, 66, 91
peer review, 100
penalties, 47
permit, 52
personal communication, 61, 62
pharmaceutical(s), 10, 80, 83, 91
physical therapist, 37
physical therapy, 15
physicians, 2, 4, 9, 13, 14, 20, 23, 24, 37, 80, 89
platform, 30

pneumonia, 11
police, 41
policy, 7, 19, 22, 30, 37, 38, 61, 63, 73, 74, 92, 93, 95
policy issues, 74
policy makers, 95
policy options, 19, 37
population, vii, 4, 6, 28, 29, 30, 32, 47, 50, 66, 75, 81, 82, 83, 88
positive interactions, 14
poverty, 28, 29
poverty line, 28
pregnancy, 30
preparedness, 29
president, v, 1, 53, 58, 59, 62, 64
prevention, 10, 94
primary function, vii
principles, vii, 4, 26, 27, 32, 33, 35, 37, 38, 87
private sector, 4, 16, 22, 25, 52, 53
problem-solving, 35, 43
process control, 9, 43
procurement, 91
product life cycle, 42
professionals, vii, 2, 4, 6, 12, 14, 24, 25, 27, 35, 37, 38, 41, 47, 62, 65, 70, 72, 78, 83, 85, 86, 92, 97, 98
profit, 4, 27, 32
profitability, 16
project, 12, 26, 33, 41, 42, 84
proliferation, 16
proteomics, 67, 83, 94
prototype, 45
public health, 31, 47, 48, 82
public interest, 48
public sector, 47
publishing, 51
pulmonary embolism, 9

## Q

quality improvement, 33, 36, 37
queuing theory, 9, 43

## R

radiation, 66, 81, 87
radiation therapy, 66, 81
radio, 87
real time, 19
recommendations, 14, 32, 38, 45, 47, 48
reengineering, 19, 27, 30
reform, 53, 57, 58, 61
registry, 21, 22
regulations, 66, 75
reimburse, 93
reliability, vii, 1, 7, 9, 18, 38, 43, 61, 90
reputation, 33
requirements, 20, 31, 32, 43, 50, 51, 66, 81, 88, 91, 95
researchers, 18, 23, 48, 51, 63, 65, 71, 72, 73, 89
residential, 21
resilience, 29
resources, 2, 10, 13, 14, 16, 19, 21, 22, 24, 27, 28, 32, 48, 52, 87, 90
response, 61
revenue, 92
rewards, 2, 15, 16
risk(s), 7, 10, 12, 16, 30, 43, 80, 81, 86, 88, 90, 91, 93, 94
risk management, 43, 91
root, 9, 85, 97
rules, 47, 80

## S

safety, vii, 4, 8, 9, 13, 25, 29, 36, 38, 52, 61, 63, 65, 70, 71, 73, 85, 86, 91, 97
scaling, 12
school, 31, 32, 36
science, 4, 9, 16, 25, 35, 36, 37, 43, 44, 52, 64, 67, 68, 72, 79, 90, 95, 98
scope, 88, 95
Secretary of Defense, 60
secure communication, 90, 92
security, 24, 46, 47
sensing, 72

# Index

sensors, 49, 100
sepsis, 11, 61
service quality, 94
services, 15, 16, 20, 24, 26, 28, 41, 42, 44, 46, 48, 49, 61, 91
shape, 98
showing, 10
simulation, 9, 77
smoking, 83
social sciences, 7, 43
social services, 29
social workers, 41
socioeconomic status, 28
software, 20, 42, 48, 49, 50, 51, 72, 76, 80
solution, 37, 39, 83
space station, 7
specialists, 12, 92, 93
spending, 70
staffing, 88
stakeholders, 4, 24, 30, 31, 32, 39, 45, 46, 47, 50, 80
standardization, 86, 87
state(s), 13, 20, 30, 33, 52, 62, 63, 69, 89, 100
statistics, 21, 70, 74
stock, 91
strategic planning, 34
stress, 10, 70
structure, 13, 26, 34, 47, 50, 69, 81, 83, 95, 100
structuring, 49, 92
substance abuse, 83
supply chain, 67, 90, 91, 92, 96
support services, 29, 41
surveillance, 24, 48
sustainability, 37
symptoms, 82
systems-engineering, vii, 1, 2, 4, 6, 7, 13, 14, 15, 19, 25, 26, 27, 30, 31, 32, 35, 37, 38, 40

## T

target, 76, 77, 82
target population(s), 82
taxonomy, 66
team members, 98
teams, 12, 28, 35, 41, 43, 64, 69, 100
technical assistance, vii, 2, 4, 14, 26, 27, 32, 38
technical support, 12, 25, 26
techniques, 2, 9, 10, 14, 33, 51, 87
technologies, 12, 52, 71, 72, 73, 76, 81, 85, 86, 91
technology, vii, 12, 18, 19, 20, 41, 44, 52, 66, 67, 68, 69, 70, 71, 72, 74, 77, 80, 82, 83, 84, 87, 88, 93, 95, 96, 97, 98, 99
technology transfer, 72
terrorism, 90
testing, 9, 11, 82, 93
threats, 85, 91
thrombosis, 9
time frame, 51
Title I, 62
Title IV, 62
Toyota, 9, 15, 42
tracks, 11
trainees, 36
training, vii, 11, 26, 27, 35, 36, 37, 85
training programs, 26
transformation, 3, 4, 17, 24, 67, 68, 83, 95, 98
translation, 51
transparency, 3, 4, 17, 23, 25, 46
transplant, 81
transportation, 28, 29, 68, 98
trauma, 9, 61
traumatic brain injury, 33
treatment, vii, 10, 15, 28, 29, 66, 81, 90, 92, 94, 95, 97

## U

U.S. Department of Commerce, 54, 64
uninsured, 29, 30, 94
United States, 45, 65, 68, 70, 74
universities, 35

## V

validation, 51
vein, 3, 9, 19
Vice President, 53, 55, 56, 58, 59
vision, 20, 35, 68, 95, 98
vocabulary, 51
volatility, 87

## W

Washington, 15, 60, 61, 62, 64

waste, 1, 9, 10, 40, 60
web, 11
wellness, 83, 94, 95
White House, 62, 64
Wisconsin, 53, 64
workers, 6
workflow, 6, 40, 49
workforce, 4, 13, 34, 37
workload, 6

## Y

yield, 81, 82, 83, 90, 91